THE
100

International
LOW-FAT
R E C I P E S

THE TOP
100

International
LOW-FAT
R E C I P E S

*Cook your weight off
easily with tasty and
easy-to-prepare dishes*

DONALD A. KULLMAN, M.D.
NANCY SZEMAN, R.D., C.D.E.

Lifetime Books, Inc.
Hollywood, Florida
800-771-3355
http: www//lifetimebooks.com
e-mail: lifetime@shadow.net

This publication is designed to provide accurate and authoritative information in regard to the subject matter covered. It is sold with the understanding
that the publisher is not engaged in rendering legal, accounting, or other professional service. If legal advice or other assistance is required, the services
of a competent professional person should be sought. *From A Declaration of
Principles jointly adopted by a Committee of the American Bar Association
and a Committee of Publishers.*

To order additional copies of *The Top 100 Low-Fat Recipes*, please send
a check or money order for $14.95 (plus $3.00 shipping/handling) to:
Lifetime Books, Inc. 2131 Hollywood Blvd., Hollywood, FL 33020.
Please write to us to receive a free catalog and information on upcoming
books that interest you.

Library of Congress Cataloging-in Publication Data
Kullman, Donald A., 1931-
     Top 100 international low-fat recipes : cook your weight off with tasty
and easy to prepare dishes / Donald A. Kullman, Nancy Szeman.
          p. cm.
     Includes index.
     ISBN 0-8119-0672-8
     1. Low-fat diet--Recipes. I. Szeman, Nancy, 1967-
II. Title.
RM237.7.K85   1996   96-32742
641.5'638 –dc20   CIP

ATTENTION READERS

This publication is designed to provide accurate and authoritative information in regard to the subject matter covered. *This book is not
intended to replace the advice and guidance of a trained physician
nor is it intended to encourage self-treatment of illness or medical
disease. Patients requiring a low-fat diet should seek counsel and
instructions from their personal physician who is familiar with their
individual case.*

Table of Contents

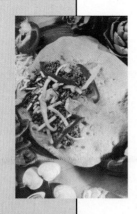

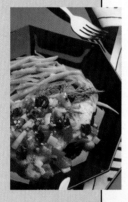
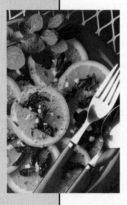

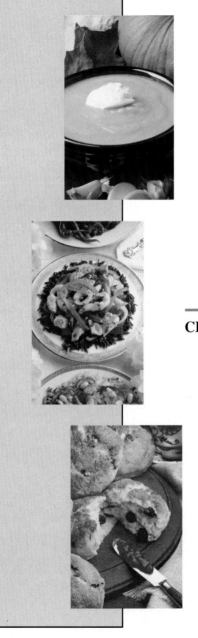

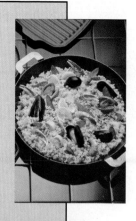

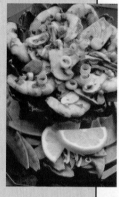

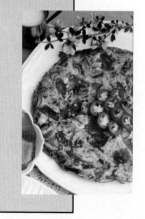

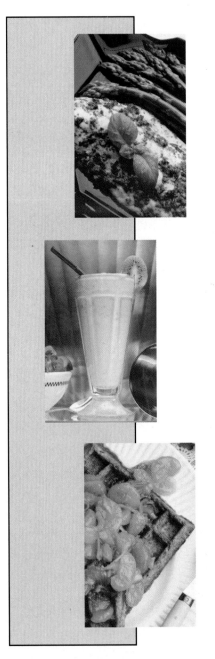

Photos by Barney Taxel

Cover by Donna Morris

Foreword

The single most important dietary change you can make to reduce your risk for cardiovascular disease — high blood pressure, heart attacks, and strokes — is to decrease the saturated fat content of your diet. An added bonus of the low- saturated-fat diet is the decline in the odds of you suffering cancer of the prostate, breast, and colon.

The American Heart Association, The American Cancer Society, The National Heart Lung and Blood Institute, as well as the surgeon general, all agree that dietary fat should be limited to 30% of the total daily caloric intake, and only one third of those fats should be of the saturated type. In other words, only 10% of daily calories should come from saturated fats. To follow these recommendations need not be difficult or complicated. Through the pages of this book the reader will be shown a simple method to stay within these guidelines.

The section on food labeling for nutritional contents will show you how to interpret the dietary information that is readily available on the nutrition fact labels of many products as now required by law. For those items that do not list their nutritional contents, the food value section of this book will serve as a convenient source for this information. Each entry is listed alphabetically with information about the caloric value of the food, the total fat, saturated fat, cholesterol, protein, carbohydrate, and sodium content. If any particular item is not listed, you can estimate its value by comparing it to a similar listed item that can serve as an approximate guide.

Following the dietary suggestions recommended in this book will help you to live not only a longer and healthier life, but will make you feel better with more vitality and energy. Weight control will be made easier because you will be consuming fewer calories even though you may be eating the same quantity of food. In short, the low-fat diet will permit you to enjoy the pleasures of eating, guilt-free.

The one hundred easy-to-prepare gourmet recipes are specially designed for everyone seeking a diet that minimizes cardiovascular risk without sacrificing the joy of eating. These recipes are proof that interesting and varied dishes are available to those who wish to take the simple steps required to insure long-term cardiovascular health. Remember, "You're only as old as your arteries." Keep them biologically young.

Are you ready, willing, and able to change your diet to improve your health? If not, you may want to ask yourself why you cannot make the effort to improve the quality of your life, because until you do so, optimal health may continue to elude you.

If you answered a firm "yes," or even if you are not quite sure, the information and diet guidance provided in this book can assist you in changing your diet to reduce your cholesterol and fat in-take and improve your health.

Ready? Good! Read through the next 250 or so pages to learn the nutritional facts and identify which foods to eat or avoid. You will soon see how simple (and tasty!) it is to eat healthfully. Whenever you dine out, use the list of dining out do's and don'ts to help you select foods wisely.

You have everything at your fingertips for beginning a new way of eating. If you choose to, if you are ready and willing, this book can enable you to eat healthfully and wisely. You can lower your blood cholesterol naturally. The choice is yours. Eat to live a long healthy life. Don't live to eat. The momentary satisfaction that rich foods offer pales in comparison with the many joys life has to offer. Don't shorten your life for a few moments of gustatory pleasure.

—Donald A Kullman, M.D.

Editor's Statement

If you are like most Americans, you want to keep excess weight off: it is better for your heart, you will look great and you will feel energetic. By reading this book you have taken a very important step to achieving all the benefits of healthy eating.

The Top 100 International Low-Fat Recipes allows you to cook your weight off with tasty and easy-to-prepare dishes. This is your comprehensive guide to preparing easy and delicious dishes that will shed fat, lower your cholesterol and help you stay fit. Now you don't have to sacrifice taste or variety for calories!

This is a unique cookbook, as it not only contains 100 ethnically diverse entree recipes, as well as 26 dessert and appetizer recipes, but it also includes: a nutritional breakdown of each recipe; a 300-item nutritional counter; a 30-day meal menu planner; a chapter on medical and health tips; and much, much more.

The Top 100 International Low-Fat Recipes will help you:
• See weight loss in just a matter of days.
• Develop and enjoy a lifetime of good habits and better health.
• Stay fit and still eat your favorite foods.

The menus featured are appetizing and creative. No single menu is repeated during the course of the month, giving more variety than most of us have at anytime. No diet pills, no starvation diets. You can lose wight and eat enjoyable meals with *The Top 100 International Low-Fat Recipes*. You can "stop the insanity" without drastically changing your lifestyle.

For more information on Lifetime Books' cookbooks, please contact us at 1-800-771-3355 or consult your favorite bookstore.

— Senior Editor
Brian Feinblum

1
Dietary Guidelines

DIET & YOUR HEART

Cardiovascular disease is currently America's number one health problem. Fortunately, there are preventative measures that you can take to increase the odds against this killing, crippling threat, even though you live in a society where much of the population will eventually suffer from heart disease, strokes, or circulatory disorders — all a result of clogged arteries laden with deposits of fat and cholesterol. Prevention of cardiovascular disease is now possible, particularly for those at high risk for cardiovascular disease. You need not become one of the victims. It is never too late to start. In some instances, the measures suggested in this book may even reverse vascular damage already sustained.

Lipids is the comprehensive term for a group of fat and fat-like substances that play a major role in the development of atherosclerosis — hardening of the arteries. Dyslipidemia (pronounced Dis-lip-id-eem-ee-uh) means abnormal levels of lipids in the blood. Cholesterol and triglycerides are the main blood lipids. Because dyslipidemia is rampant in the United

States as a consequence of the typical American high-saturated-fat diet, perhaps as many as half of the population has dangerously high cholesterol levels and are at significant risk for developing cardiovascular disease.

The corrective steps required to insure cardiovascular health depend on a number of factors, some of which are under your control, others are unchangeable. To evaluate your predisposition to cardiovascular disease, the following simple self-test will enable you to score how your present life style promotes cardiovascular health.

CARDIOVASCULAR RISK ASSESSMENT SELF-TEST

Yes	No	Unsure	
___	___	___	1. I have a family history of high blood pressure, heart disease,circulatory disorders, and/or stroke.
___	___	___	2. I have diabetes.
___	___	___	3. I smoke cigarettes.
___	___	___	4. I do not exercise regularly.
___	___	___	5. I am often tense and feel stressed.
___	___	___	6. I have a high blood cholesterol level (over 200).
___	___	___	7. I have high blood pressure (above 140/90).
___	___	___	8. I am overweight.

If you answered "no" to all of these statements, your risk of developing cardiovascular disease is not great. You lifestyle is "heart healthy." However, the more "yes" responses you gave, the more likely your lifestyle predisposes you to strokes, heart attacks, or circulatory disorders.

This Self-Test actually illustrates the important "risk factors" which are believed to contribute to the development of cardiovascular disease. By controlling these risk factors, it may be possible for you to reduce your chances of ever having a heart attack, stroke, or circulatory disorder.

RISK FACTORS

The eight major risk factors are :
- family history of cardiovascular disease
- diabetes
- cigarette smoking
- physical inactivity
- hyperlipidemia — high blood levels of cholesterol and triglycerides
- hypertension — high blood pressure
- obesity
- age — above 45 yrs. in males — over 55 yrs. in females (not taking estrogen replacement therapy)

Your susceptibility to cardiovascular disease may have been programmed into your genes before you were born. But what does it really mean to have inherited a family tendency for heart disease? A family history for coronary artery disease (particularly a family history of heart attacks before age 55) means that degenerative changes in the coronary arteries may occur at an accelerated rate, resulting in the appearance of cardiovascular disease at a relatively young age. What is inherited is the genetic programming for the way your body metabolizes fats and cholesterol. The main culprit that causes the chain of events that over time damage the blood vessel walls and leads to a heart attack or stroke, is a chronically elevated blood cholesterol level.

The relationship between the cholesterol level and heart disease does not abruptly change at any particular level. Rather there is a continuous lowering of cardiovascular disease risk as the level declines. In general, each 1% drop in cholesterol is accompanied by a 2% decline in heart disease. For some persons, particularly those with multiple risk factors, the so-called normal upper limit of cholesterol may still be too high.

An example that clearly demonstrates the importance of diet on the incidence and death rate from cardiovascular disease is the analysis of data from pre and post-war Europe. Before the war, heart attacks were not uncommon among Europeans. During the war, meat, milk, eggs, and other sources of saturated fat and cholesterol were scarce. People survived on simple grains and vegetables. As the population became lean on its imposed low fat diet, cholesterol levels fell and the rate of heart attacks and strokes dropped dramatically. With peace and post-war prosperity, the population returned to its pre-war eating habits. The rate of cardiovascular diseases once more climbed to pre-war levels.

Fat Metabolism

To understand the undesirable vascular changes related to diet and their prevention, it is necessary to have a basic knowledge of the body's fat metabolism. Lipids is the comprehensive term for a group of fat and fat-like substances that play a major role in the development of arteriosclerosis, the general term for thickening and hardening of the arteries. Atherosclerosis is a type of arteriosclerosis characterized by the deposit of fatty substances, cholesterol, cellular waste products, calcium and fibrin (a blood substance that plays an important role in the blood clotting mechanism) in the inner lining of the blood vessels. The resultant build-up is called plaque.

Although cholesterol has become a household word, much confusion remains regarding this waxy, fat-like substance. Perhaps no other element in our diet has been the source of such intense controversy. However, the jury is no longer out; a verdict has been rendered. Case closed. The Framingham epidemiological study of more than 5000 men and women over a twenty-five year period clearly demonstrated the link between elevated cholesterol and heart disease. The other major risk factors, as already noted, include cigarette smoking, sedentary lifestyle, high blood pressure, obesity, diabetes and family history for cardiovascular events.

Cholesterol is a soft fat-like substance that is vital for performing a number of essential biological functions including making cell membranes, sex hormones and the sheaths that cover nerve fibers. To meet these needs, "Mother Nature" has provided for the liver to manufacture adequate amounts of cholesterol. Typically, the body makes all the cholesterol it needs. There is no daily dietary requirement for cholesterol — it is not necessary to consume any to maintain health.

Although cholesterol is found only in products of animal origin, saturated fats, whether derived from animal or vegetable products, stimulate the liver to produce cholesterol. In fact, they act as the raw material for cholesterol production. Saturated fats in the diet play an even greater role than dietary cholesterol in raising blood cholesterol levels. The other types of dietary fat are called "polyunsaturated fats" and "monosaturated fats." These, along with Omega 3 fatty acids, may have a beneficial effect on lipid levels and do not raise cholesterol — more about this later.

"Oil and water don't mix." Body fluids, blood, serum and lymph, are all water based. Lipids are not soluble in water. For lipids to enter the body fluids and be transported throughout the body, they must link up with proteins forming compounds called lipoproteins. The protein is the transport vehicle and the lipid is the cargo.

CHOLESTEROL CIRCULATION

There are two major types of lipoproteins involved in the transport of cholesterol. Low density lipoproteins (LDL) and high density lipoproteins (HDL). The LDL (LDL-Cholesterol) delivers the cholesterol to the body's cells. However, when there is an excess amount of cholesterol, the surplus may be deposited on the walls of the blood vessels forming the scarred areas called plaques. Thus begins the atherosclerotic process that can eventually choke and clog the artery. For this reason LDL is sometimes called "Bad Cholesterol." The HDL-cholesterol removes excess cholesterol from the blood and new evidence suggests that it sometimes extracts it from existing plaque deposits as well, carrying it back to the liver where it can be re-used or broken down and excreted. HDL is therefore known as "Good Cholesterol."

PLAQUE

If LDL-cholesterol remains elevated through the years, it may cause the opening of the blood vessel to gradually narrow as plaque deposits encroach on the lumen. When the vessel is completely occluded, the tissue beyond the point of obstruction loses its blood supply. The narrowing of the blood vessel by plaque deposits need not be complete to cause a serious health threat. In fact, microscopic size areas of damage to the inner lining of the blood vessel can represent a major health threat. Hemorrhage into the plaque or rupture of the plaque may cause sudden death. Plaque causes the inner lining of the blood vessel to lose its smooth contour.

Small eddy currents may form as the blood passes over the uneven lining of the damaged blood vessel. This disturbance in the blood flow favors the formation of a blood clot. Unless there is some collateral circulation, the tissue that depended on that blood vessel for its life sustaining functions dies. When this process occurs in one of the arteries that supplies the heart muscle itself — a coronary artery — the result is called a "coronary thrombosis," or "heart attack." If the same process takes place in one of the blood vessels in the brain, the resultant condition is called a "stroke."

BLOOD CLOTTING

For the blood clotting mechanism to begin, certain particles that normally circulate in the blood, called platelets, are required. The clotting process is initiated when the platelets become sticky and adhere to one another and the blood vessel wall. Ordinary aspirin has the effect of preventing this platelet stickiness from developing. Aspirin, in low doses, effectively reduces the risk of heart attacks. The dose of aspirin required is small. Too large a dose has a paradoxical effect, and does not afford protection. One baby aspirin daily suffices. Enteric coated 80mg aspirin, equivalent to a baby aspirin tablet, are now available and reduce the risk of gastric irritation that may be seen with plain aspirin.

Despite a declining death rate from many causes, coronary artery disease still ranks as the number one killer in America. This is particularly true not only for those over the age of 65, but also for men in the 45-65 year-old age group. As one would suspect, middle-aged men with coronary artery disease are generally found to have significantly higher levels of cholesterol and triglycerides than those without heart disease.

It has long been known that diabetics are prone to developing atherosclerosis and heart disease about ten to twelve years earlier than the population at large. The dyslipidemia that accompanies diabetes is an integral part of the disorder because diabetes is a disturbance of lipid metabolism as well as carbohydrate metabolism.

The medical guidelines for classifying blood cholesterol levels advise that a total cholesterol level of less than 200mg/dl is "desirable" for adults. There are three categories of total cholesterol:

Total Cholesterol Categories:

Desirable Blood Cholesterol	Borderline-High Blood Cholesterol	High Blood Cholesterol
less than 200mg/dl	200-239mg/dl	240mg/dl and above

Cholesterol levels less than 200mg/dl are considered desirable, while levels of 240mg/dl or above are high and require more specific attention. Levels from 200-239 mg/dl also require attention, especially if the HDL-cholesterol is low or LDL level is high or if there are two or more other risk factors for heart disease.

LDL-Cholesterol

Desirable	Borderline-High Risk	High Risk
less than 130mg/dl	130-159mg/dl	above 160mg/dl

The LDL level gives a better picture of the risk for heart disease than the total cholesterol level. Accordingly, most physicians consider lowering LDL as the main treatment goal for a cholesterol problem. If your LDL level puts you at high-risk and you have fewer than two other risk factors for heart disease, your target goal should be an LDL level of less than 160mg/dl. However, if you have two or more other risk factors for heart disease, your LDL goal should be less than 130mg/dl. If you already have heart disease, your LDL target should be even lower — 100mg/dl or less. These target goals suggested by The National Cholesterol Educational Program (NCEP), may be summarized as follows:

THE NCEP RECOMMENDATIONS

For individuals with:	Initiate drug therapy* if LDL cholesterol is:	LDL cholesterol goal is:
No coronary heart disease (CHD) and fewer than two other CHD risk factors	≥ 190 mg/dL after ≥ 6 months of diet	<160 mg/dL
No CHD but with two or more other CHD risk factors	≥ 160 mg/dL after ≥ 6 months of diet	<130 mg/dL
Definite CHD or other atherosclerotic disease	≥ 130 mg/dL after 6-12 weeks of Step II diet	≤ 100 mg/dL

*Following an adequate trial of diet.

National Cholesterol Education Program: Second report of the Expert Panel on Detection, Evaluation, and Treatment of High Blood Cholesterol in Adults (Adult Treatment Panel II), NIH Publication No. 93-3095, Bethesda, MD, National Heart, Lung, and Blood Institute, September 1993.

Your doctor should look at all your risk factors to decide what measures to take to lower your blood cholesterol and reduce your risk of heart disease.

HDL-CHOLESTEROL

Normal HDL	Low HDL	High HDL
more than 35 mg/dl	less than 35mg/dl	above 60 mg/dl

Unlike total cholesterol and LDL-cholesterol, the lower your HDL, the higher your risk for heart disease. An HDL level less than 35mg/dl is considered low and increases your risk for heart disease. The higher your HDL, the better. An HDL level of 60mg/dl or above is high and is associated with longevity. Alcohol raises the HDL. However, the chemical fraction of the HDL elevated by alcohol is not the portion of HDL cholesterol that is protective against atherosclerosis. Therefore, high HDL levels in alcoholics can give a distorted view of the significance of this finding. An HDL level below 35 is considered a risk factor. An HDL over 60 usually is protective — a negative risk factor. HDL levels are particularly effective in their protective action in females. It is therefore probably fair to place more weight on the significance of levels of HDL-cholesterol in women than in men.

CHOLESTEROL/HDL RATIO

The importance of the level of total cholesterol can be determined only after evaluation of the types of cholesterol that contribute to the total reading. A frequently simplified formula that yields practical information is the ration of total cholesterol to HDL-cholesterol.

A total cholesterol level of 260mg% may have entirely different significance for two individuals with different lipid metabolism. If the HDL level is high, the ratio may be within normal limits and not represent a health threat despite the high total cholesterol level. If the HDL were low, the elevated cholesterol would require management. Even though the general guidelines state that a cholesterol level below 200mg% is desirable, if an individual with a low total cholesterol reading has a low HDL level, the ratio would be high and indicate vulnerability to cardiovascular disease. Conversely, as noted, an individual with a high total cholesterol, with a high HDL-cholesterol, might well have a satisfactory total cholesterol/HDL ratio and not be at risk for cardiovascular disease. The following reference values can serve as a general guide:

Coronary Heart Disease Risk*	_Total Cholesterol/HDL Ratio_	
	Male	Female
1/2 Average	3.4	3.3
Average (normal)	5.0	4.4
Twice Average (moderate)	9.6	7.0
Three Times Average (high)	13.4	11.0

* Data based on Framingham Study

TRIGLYCERIDES

Triglycerides are fats that circulate in the blood and serve as energy sources. Based on your age, your triglyceride levels should not rise above the following:

AGE	INCREASED RISK
19-29	> 140mg/dl
30-39	> 150
40-49	> 160
> 49	> 190

Triglyceride levels must be done on blood obtained after an overnight fast of at least 14 hours, otherwise erroneously high levels may result. Total cholesterol levels may be performed on non-fasting blood. HDL-cholesterol levels, however, must be done on fasting specimens for accurate results.

If both total cholesterol levels and triglycerides are elevated, it will be necessary to not only limit the saturated fats in your diet, but the simple sugars, alcohol and fruits as well. Vegetables may be eaten freely.

MEASURES TO REDUCE DYSLIPIDEMIA

Dyslipidemia that cannot be brought under control by careful management of diet, weight reduction, and adequate exercise calls for a search for "secondary" causes of the abnormal lipid levels (i.e. hypothyroidism, genetic hypercholesterolemia, kidney or liver disease, alcoholism, diabetes etc.). If these "secondary" causes of dyslipidemia are "ruled out," and diet cannot yield satisfactory control, drug therapy must be considered by the physician to aid in reducing the blood lipids.

The National Cholesterol Education Adult Treatment Panel recommended target goals for LDL-cholesterol that can often only be achieved with the aid of cholesterol lowering medications. However, the first step in the treatment of elevated total cholesterol and LDL levels is diet. As noted, The American Heart Association's "Prudent Diet," recommends that total fat intake should be no more than 30% of daily caloric dietary intake and only 1/3 of that fat should be of the saturated type. A more aggressive approach to lowering cholesterol is taken by the Pritikin Program, which restricts total fat intake to 10% of the daily caloric value with the majority of those fats in the unsaturated form. Most people are unwilling to make the stringent dietary changes demanded by the Pritikin Program. For those willing to do so the rewards can be substantial. For more information, you may write to the Pritikin Longevity Center, 1910 Ocean Front Walk, Santa Monica, CA 90405-1014.

DIETARY MEASURES TO LOWER CHOLESTEROL

The typical American diet is outrageously high in saturated fats. Dairy products, fried foods, pastries, hot dogs, hamburgers, and pizzas are but a few examples of foods extremely high in cholesterol and saturated fats. Even a lean filet mignon with no visible streaking has at least 30% fat content! It should come

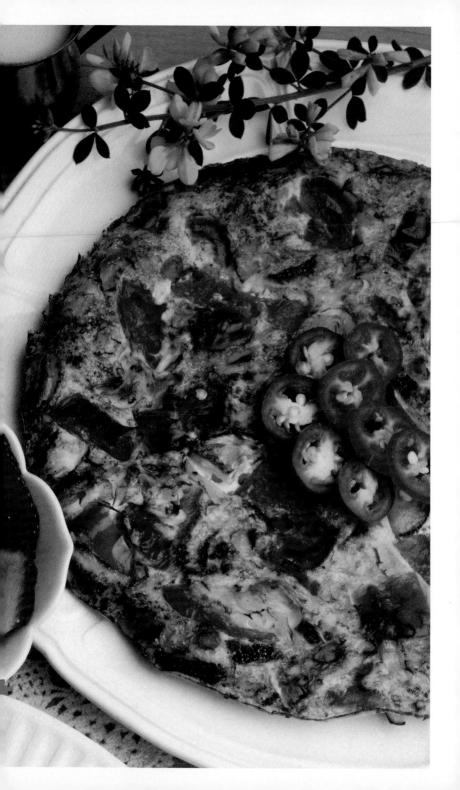

Italian-Style Frittata
A low-cholesterol alternative for breakfast, lunch or dinner.

Photo Credits
Photography by Barney Taxel
Barney Taxel & Co.
216/431-2400

Recipe Credits
Italian-Style Frittata, see page 127
Servings: 4

as no surprise that heart disease has reached epidemic proportions in this country.

Now that you know about blood cholesterol, get set to lower it. Everyone, regardless of his blood cholesterol level, should eat in a heart-healthy way. This is true beginning with toddlers (about age 2) on up to their parents, grandparents, and even great-grandparents. The whole family should also be physically active. If you have a high blood cholesterol level — whether due to what you eat or to heredity — it is even more important to eat healthfully and to be physically active. Adopting these measures also can help control high blood pressure as well as diabetes. Following a low fat diet can reduce your cholesterol about 15%. In general, the greater the saturated fat restriction, the lower the cholesterol.

HERE ARE SOME GENERAL DIETARY RULES TO LOWER BLOOD CHOLESTEROL:

Choose Foods Low In Saturated Fat

All foods that contain fat are made up of a mixture of saturated and unsaturated fats. Saturated fat raises your blood cholesterol level more than anything else that you eat. It is found in greatest amounts in foods from animal sources, such as fatty cuts of meat, poultry with the skin, whole-milk dairy products, lard, as well as in some vegetable oils like coconut, palm kernel, and palm oils. These latter oils, high in saturated fats, often hide behind the food label "non-dairy." They are frequently used in processed foods — commercial baked goods, fried snacks, and non-dairy toppings and cream substitutes. Don't fall into the nondairy trap. Read food labels carefully. The best way to reduce your blood cholesterol level is to select foods low in saturated fat. One way to do this is by choosing foods such as fruits, vegetables, whole grain foods, including breads and cereals naturally low in fat and high in starch and fiber.

Since many foods high in saturated fat are also high in total fat, eating foods low in saturated fat will help you eat less total fat. When you do eat fat, you should substitute unsaturated fat for saturated fat. Unsaturated fat is usually liquid at room temperature and can be either monosaturated or polyunsaturated. Examples of foods high in monosaturated fat are olive and canola oils (Puritan®). Those high in polyunsaturated fat, include safflower, sunflower, corn, and soybean oils. Any type of fat is a rich source of calories, so eating foods low in fat will also help you to keep your weight under control.

DIET CURES: THE UN-FATS

Monosaturated fats can help to lower total blood cholesterol without lowering HDL-cholesterol. Due to this discovery, physicians and nutritionists now recommend cooking with canola oil (Puritan®) or olive oil and using olive oil on salads when desired.

The important role of "omega-3 fatty acids" in human health is often overlooked. This type of unsaturated fat contributes to a reduced risk of cardiovascular disease, as diets rich in omega-3's help to lower blood cholesterol levels, reduce blood pressure and clotting, and inhibit atherosclerosis. The omega-3 fatty acids are abundant in fatty cold water fish, but are also found in lean fish and other marine life, including shellfish. Evidence points to an omega-3 fatty acid called eicosapentaenoic acid (EPA) as the chief protective agent against heart disease. Eating only two fish dishes per week may offer protection against heart disease. The omega-3 fatty acids should be obtained from natural food sources only. Capsule supplements of these substances have been implicated in causing untoward side effects.

As noted, by reducing total fat intake, you can help to lower your cholesterol level. Select foods from the two lists that follow, the MONO-FAT FOODS LIST and the OMEGA-3 FOODS LIST, to partially replace the saturated fats in your diet. For example, substitute a broiled fish dinner for red meats several times a week. Stir-fry vegetables in canola or olive oil, and use olive oil in tomato sauce and other dishes. Indulge in shellfish, like crab or scallops. Even though they have some cholesterol, they are low in saturated fats. Your heart, if not your wallet, can afford it!

Mono-Fat Foods List

almonds	filberts (hazelnuts)	peanuts
avocados	olives	pecans
cashews	olive oil	seafood

Omega-3 Foods List
Richest Sources

anchovies	fresh water trout	mackerel
bass	halibut	salmon
bluefish	herring	tuna

Also Good Omega-3 Sources

clams	haddock	scallops
cod	lobster	shrimp
crab	mussels	swordfish
flounder	oysters	other cold water fish

CHOOSE FOODS HIGH IN STARCH & FIBER

Foods high in starch and fiber are excellent substitutes for foods high in saturated fat. These foods — whole wheat breads, cereals, pasta, grains (such as oats and barley), dry peas, beans, fruits, and vegetables — are low in saturated fat and contain no cholesterol. They are also usually lower in calories than foods that are high in fat, as well as being good sources of vitamins and minerals.

CHOOSE FOODS LOW IN CHOLESTEROL

Dietary cholesterol also can raise your blood cholesterol level, although usually not as much as saturated fat. Although this generality is true, individual metabolic pathways, for handling dietary cholesterol, vary from person to person. Some individuals may eat foods high in cholesterol without any significant adverse effects on their blood cholesterol levels. However, for most people, it is recommended to choose foods low in cholesterol. Dietary cholesterol is found only in foods that come from animals. Many of these foods are also high in saturated fat, so by avoiding high cholesterol foods, you will be cutting back on saturated fats which play the major role in raising blood cholesterol. Foods from plant sources do not have cholesterol but can contain saturated fat. The main plant sources of fats are avocados, olives, palm oil and coconut oil, with only the latter two being mainly of the saturated fat type.

CHOLESTEROL IN FOODS

A prudent diet minimizes high cholesterol foods, notably egg yolks, organ meats, fatty meats, such as bacon and burgers, butter, cream, and whole milk products. The suggested daily maximum cholesterol intake is 300mg. Many physicians consider this level too high and limit their patients to 200mg/day. A single egg yolk contains some 280mg. The white of the egg is fat and cholesterol-free. The prudent diet limits eggs to one or two per week. Organ meats (liver, kidney, and sweetbreads) should be eaten no more than once a month or preferably not at all. Other high-cholesterol foods (see list below) can be avoided entirely, or eaten in limited amounts on occasion, if desired. The choice is yours.

High Cholesterol Foods List

bacon
burgers
butter
caviar
cheese (unless low-fat)
cold cuts
cream
cream cheese
egg yolk

eggnog
fatty meat (choice, marbled, and prime cuts; spareribs)
hot dogs
ice cream
lard
milk, whole; half & half
organ meats (kidney, liver)
slat pork, sausages
sour cream, whipped cream

Sources of Saturated Fat and Cholesterol

Animal fat
Bacon fat
Beef fat
Butter
Chicken fat
Cocoa butter
Coconut
Coconut oil ***
Cream
Egg and egg yolk solids
Ham fat

Hardened fat or oil*
Lamb fat
Lard
Meat fat
Palm kernel oil
Pork fat
Turkey fat
Vegetable oil**
Vegetable shortening
Whole milk solids

* Hiding behind the label "partially hydrogenated vegetable oil." Hydrogenation is the chemical process that transforms oils that are unsaturated and liquid at room temperature, to a more solid and saturated state. This process increases the

shelf life of the product and helps to retain fresh flavor. It is therefore a favorite of commercial bakers. The label "partially hydrogenated" vegetable oil really means "partially saturated fat".

** Could be coconut or palm oil.

*** Often used in non-dairy cream substitutes, some frozen deserts, and cocoa butter in chocolate.

Be More Physically Active

Being physically active helps your blood cholesterol levels: Exercise can raise HDL and may lower LDL. Being more active also can help you lose weight, lower your blood pressure, improve the fitness of your heart and blood vessels, and reduce stress.

Lose Weight, If You Are Overweight

People who are overweight tend to have higher blood cholesterol levels than people of desirable weight. When you cut the fat in your diet, you cut down on the richest source of calories. An eating pattern high in starch and fiber instead of fat is a good way to lose weight.

Starchy foods have little fat and ounce for ounce are lower in calories than high fat foods. If you are overweight, losing even a little weight can help to lower LDL-cholesterol and raise HDL-cholesterol. You do not need to wait until you reach your desirable weight to see a change in your blood cholesterol levels.

Review : To Lower Your Blood Cholesterol, Remember To:
- Choose foods low in saturated fat and cholesterol.
- Be more physically active
- Lose weight, if you are overweight.

CHOLESTEROL-LOWERING DRUG
THERAPY FOR DYSLIPIDEMIA

Regardless of the factors contributing to your high cholesterol, diet still remains the keystone measure to correct this condition. However, there are many persons who follow a strict low-fat , low-cholesterol diet, who are still unable to lower their cholesterol. Others may eat whatever they wish, including saturated fats, and enjoy normal lipid levels. These lucky rare individuals need not concern themselves with dietary fat restrictions.

For most people, however, if persistent and faithful dietary measures prove inadequate to achieve target goals, medications are available that can lower cholesterol and triglyceride levels. An important advance in recent years has been the development of a new class of cholesterol-lowering drugs.

HMG-CoA Reductase Inhibitors: The introduction of a new class of cholesterol-lowering drugs that work by interfering with the synthesis of cholesterol has revolutionized the treatment of dyslipidemia. The HMG-CoA reductase inhibitors, or "statins," have heralded a new era of treatment for hypercholesterolemia. Included in this category of drugs are Lovastatin (Mevacor®), Simvastatin (Zocor®), Fluvastatin (Lescol®), and Pravastatin (Pravachol®): These pharmacological agents have proven to be safe, well tolerated and very effective. Given in appropriate doses under medical supervision, this class of drugs has been shown in will documented studies to significantly lower the incidence of cardiovascular disease.

Unique to pravastatin (Pravachol®) therapy is the potential benefit of preventing acute coronary artery events (heart attacks and unstable angina) as early as six months to one year after instituting therapy. This short period of time for therapeutic effect may result from a physiological action independent of its cholesterol lowering properties. It has been theorized that this early protective benefit may be a result of stabilization of existing plaques as well as some, still as yet poorly understood biological alterations in the blood vessel wall.

It is believed that the stability of plaques and the condition of the inner lining of the blood vessel play major roles in acute coronary events. Plaque rupture explains the not infrequent acute coronary events in those with minor plaque formation (less than 30% occlusion of a coronary artery). This phenomenon would also explain the sudden deaths in asymptomatic individuals who have an apparently normal electrocardiogram without clinical evidence of cardiovascular disease.

In short, stabilization of small plaques and improvement in the function of the blood vessel lining may explain this important early protective benefit of Pravachol® as a phenomenon beyond its blood cholesterol lowering effect. Small asymptomatic plaque lesions are responsible for more than 80% of acute coronary events.

In November 1994, the 5 year Scandinavian Simvastin Survival Study (known as the 4 S Study) provided a controlled scientific look at more than 4000 men who had either survived a heart attack or had angina pectoris (coronary insufficiency). The cholesterol level of the subjects averaged 260mg/dl. The study had a double-blind, placebo controlled format. The participants were divided into two groups. Half of them received simvastatin and the other half were given placebo pills. The results clearly demonstrated the benefits of lowering blood cholesterol levels with medication. Those receiving the cholesterol lowering drugs had a much lower incidence of coronary by-pass surgery or balloon angiography, surgical treatments indicated for advanced coronary artery disease.

The overall mortality within the treated group was 30% less than in the control group. In other words, not only did far fewer patients require surgical intervention for advanced coronary disease, but the improved lipid level was accompanied by an overall improvement in health and decreased mortality.

In November 1995, Dr. James Shepherd of the University of Glasgow, reported the results of the landmark Pravachol Primary Prevention Study (also known as The West of Scotland Coronary Prevention Study), in the prestigious New England Journal of Medicine (Sheppherd, 1995). This double-blind, four year study involved more than 6500 Scottish men, aged 45-64, with cholesterol levels of 250-300mg/dl with no known heart disease who were treated with pravastatin.

The results far exceeded the anticipated benefits of even the most optimistic proponents of drug intervention. The treated group had 33% fewer heart attacks, 20% fewer deaths from all causes, and 20% fewer by-pass surgical procedures. The importance of treating a large segment of the population that has no known heart disease, but does have elevated cholesterol levels, was clearly demonstrated by the West of Scotland Study.

The study showed that drug intervention should be resorted to earlier than previously believed. If diet and exercise cannot achieve satisfactory reduction in abnormal lipid levels, drug therapy is definitely indicated. Those with additional risk factors are particularly vulnerable. These are the asymptomatic individuals with silent underlying cardiovascular disease who may die without warning symptoms.

Cardiologist Dr. Eugene Braunwald, of Harvard and Boston's, Brigham and Women's Hospital, is quite emphatic in his recommendations for the use of these drugs. "We're talking about a therapeutic revolution", Dr. Braunwald told a recent gathering of the American Heart Association in Orlando, Florida.

Patients on the "statins" must be monitored by their physician for adverse side effects such as elevated liver enzymes. In general, however, this class of drugs is well tolerated. The side effects are usually mild and reversible. Blood tests to monitor liver function should be done periodically. Muscle inflammation, called myopathy, has been seen in less than one half of one percent of those on these medications.

The goal of all Americans should be to prevent heart attacks and preserve their cardiovascular health. Don't wait until you have a heart attack to stop smoking and make changes in your lifestyle and eating habits. Playing catch-up is much more difficult than taking the simple preventive measures now recommended by all of the experts in the field. Survivors of heart attacks are not home free. Many are forced to cope with a decreased quality of life.

As noted, with the loss of the protective effect of estrogens after menopause, the incidence of cardiovascular disease in post-menopausal women gradually rises until it approximates that of their male counterparts. Estrogen replacement therapy is of value in reducing coronary artery disease in women in this age group, if there are no medical contraindications to its use as determined by a physician.

Some elevation of the HDL-cholesterol can be accomplished by weight loss and exercise. The use of moderate amounts of alcohol daily, two drinks per day, seems to help prevent heart disease. **More than 2 drinks has a harmful effect on lipids. If you don't drink — don't start.** The French paradox is the phenomenon seen in France where a large segment of the population drinks red wine and eats high cholesterol foods without undo risk for heart disease.

Dietary Guidelines for Limiting Fat Intake

As already emphasized, the major dietary culprit for high blood cholesterol levels is the saturated fat content of the diet. The American Heart Association "Prudent Diet" recommends limiting total daily fat intake to 30% of daily caloric needs, of which no more than 1/3 is to be in the form of saturated fat. The remaining 20% will therefore be unsaturated fats — either monosaturated or polyunsaturated — 300mg cholesterol/ day is permitted. These recommendations represent an improvement over the typical American diet and have played a major role in the decline of heart disease seen over the past twenty years, as a large segment of the population heeded these dietary guidelines.

The Pritikin Program limits total fat intake to 10% of daily caloric needs, with most of those fat calories coming from unsaturated fats. Cholesterol is restricted to less than 100mg/ day. Highly motivated individuals who are willing to live by the stringent Pritikin guidelines may well reap a reward that will make the effort worthwhile.

If you wish to pursue the Pritikin route, you can get additional information in any of the books published by the Pritikin Institute. If you feel you need professional monitoring and guidance, the Pritikin Centers offer resident programs where you get the benefits of a controlled environment with professional supervision.

FOLLOWING THE RECOMMENDED GUIDELINES MADE EASY

How to Estimate the Quantities of Saturated Fat in Foods that Represent 10% of Daily Caloric Intake

The following caloric estimates are offered only as approximate general guidelines to calculate daily caloric requirements. Assuming average physical activity and age 20-35, the average male requires 15cal/lb of body weight/day. After age 35, there is a gradual decline in caloric needs as metabolism declines with age. At age 65 a male might require only 13-14cal/ lb to meet daily needs. A very active physical life will require more calories to maintain body weight. A sedentary lifestyle will need fewer calories. For example, a male subject, 30 years of age, weight 150 lbs., whose lifestyle involves average physical activity, would require approximately 2250 calories/day (weight in pounds x 15cal/lb — 150 x 15 = 2250cal/day). If he is physically quite active he might need 2800 calories. If his lifestyle is sedentary, 1900 calories might suffice. To determine the amount of calories derived from saturated fat that are permitted (10% of the total calories allowed), merely shift the decimal point to the left. For example, if 2250 calories is the daily intake allowed, no more than 225 calories should come from saturated fat. Inasmuch as all fats yield 9 calories per gram, we have only to divide the 225 calories by 9 to determine the number of grams of fat that will supply the number of saturated fat calories permitted. In this case, 225 divided by 9 yields 25 grams. The following chart shows at a glance the grams of saturated fat permitted for various caloric levels.

Amount of saturated fat permitted

Caloric Needs	10% From Saturated Fat
1000 calories	11 grams
1200 calories	13 grams
1500 calories	17 grams
2000 calories	22 grams
2500 calories	23 grams
3000 calories	33 grams

Inasmuch as polyunsaturated fats do not raise blood cholesterol and monosaturated fat seem to have a cholesterol protective effect, we need only concern ourselves with dietary saturated fats.

READ FOOD LABELS

Read the nutrition information and look at the ingredients

Learning how to interpret the data on food labels will help you choose foods low in saturated fat, cholesterol, calories, and sodium. What will the labels tell you? Food labels have two important parts: the nutrition information and the ingredients list. Also, some labels have different claims like "low fat" or "light." Generally, low-fat foods must have a fat content of ten percent or less. However, these terms are not standardized and have little meaning. Here's a closer look at labels.

Look for the amount of saturated fat, total fat, cholesterol, and calories in a serving of a product. Compare similar products to find the one with the smallest amounts. If you have high blood pressure, do the same for sodium, particularly if you are 45 years of age or older. All food labels list the product's ingredients in order by weight. The ingredient in the greatest amount is listed first. To determine the saturated fat content of foods in grams you have only to read the quantity of saturated fat in grams listed under that heading. For those items that do not have nutritional labels, the Food Value Section of this book will serve as a convenient source for this information. You can estimate the value of non-listed items by comparing them to similar items that can serve as an approximate guide.

The recipes described in this book yield tasty dishes equally as satisfying as their more fatty counterparts. Many of the common offending high fat foods have been replaced with non-fat equivalents of excellent palatability. Non-fat sour cream is now available that is both tasty and similar in texture to its fatty counterpart. Even ground beef may be replaced with Boca Burgers® , derived completely from vegetable products. When prepared with condiments, this substitute compares favorably with the high fat American staple — the hamburger. The cholesterol content of eggs, liver and sweet breads is quite high. Eggs can be replaced with egg replacers available in most supermarkets, or three whites of the egg may be used to replace two whole eggs. The yolk is the source of the cholesterol and fat.

PRODUCT: **CHECK FOR:**

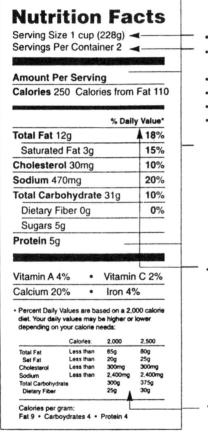

- Serving size
- Number of servings

- Calories
- Total fat in grams
- Saturated fat in grams
- Cholesterol in milligrams

Here, the label gives the amounts for the different nutrients in one serving. Use it to help you keep track of how much fat, saturated fat, cholesterol, and calories you are getting from different foods.

- The "% Daily Value" shows you how much of the recommended amounts the food provides in one serving, if you eat 2,000 calories a day. For example, one serving of this food gives you 18 percent of your total fat recommendation.

- Here you can see the recommended daily amounts for each nutrient for two calorie levels. If you eat a 2,000 calorie diet, you should be eating less than 65 grams of fat and less than 20 grams of saturated fat. Your daily amounts may vary higher or lower depending on your calorie needs.

Obesity

The human body is a machine. If we ingest more calories than we expend, the excess is converted into fat and stored. If we use more calories than we ingest, we borrow from our fat reserves and we lose weight. To lose one pound per week requires a decreased caloric intake of 500 calories per day or 3500 calories per week. In short, obesity is caused by taking in too many calories or by not expending enough energy to burn up the caloric content of the diet that exceeds the body's requirements, or a combination of both of these factors. Additional elements that are more obscure, but that have been shown to play important roles in obesity are as follows:

1. Genetic alterations in the "appetite control center" (in the hypothalamic area of the brain).
2. The level of fat in the diet. Calorie for calorie, fat calories will make you fatter than proteins or carbohydrates because of the way the body metabolizes fat. In other words, weight loss is facilitated by diets low in fat even though the caloric intake may be the same as a comparable diet with higher fat content.
3. Eating patterns can contribute to obesity. Skipping breakfast and consuming most of the daily calories with the evening meal can lead to weight gain. People who skip meals burn fewer calories than those who divide their caloric intake into three or more separate meals.
4. Chronic dieting! The metabolic rate declines with weight loss, making the task of shedding weight more difficult the longer one is on a diet. When the patient resumes his regular diet, weight gain actually occurs easier than before because chronic dieting has been shown to lead to a reduction in basal metabolic rate. Chronically dieting people have basal metabolic rates 10-20% below normal.

Data from the National Health and Nutrition Examination Survey substantiated the claim of many obese people who insist they do not eat more than their lean counterparts.

5. Obesity. Obese people tend to be less active than non-obese people. If caloric intake remains unchanged, increased activity or exercise is the only way to lose weight. Modest increases in physical activity seem to suppress appetite. However, marked increases of physical activity seem to stimulate appetite and caloric intake, although usually not to the extent of the additional calories expended.

6. Aging and accompanying inactivity. Basal metabolic caloric requirements gradually decrease with age, although appetite may remain unchanged. A continued unchanged caloric intake without the physical activity and exercise required to burn this excess fuel tips the balance towards obesity.

Being overweight is not only unattractive, it is hazardous to your health! Excess poundage can contribute to:

- decreased respiratory function and sleep apnea.
- type II diabetes (adult onset)
- gallbladder disorders
- infertility
- chronic joint pain and arthritis (osteoarthritis and gout)
- certain types of cancer including breast, prostate, and colon cancer
- cardiovascular disease (heart attacks & strokes)
- high blood pressure
- varicose veins
- elevated blood cholesterol
- decreased longevity

Weight reduction has been shown to reduce high blood pressure and high blood cholesterol levels, improving blood lipid

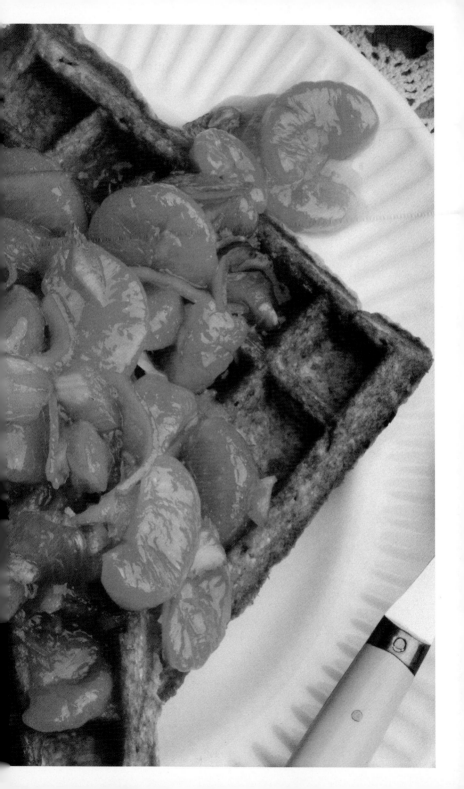

Oat Bran & Apple Waffle with Apricots

High in fiber, high in flavor! Try this low-fat delight as an alternative to heavy desserts.

Photo Credits

Photography by Barney Taxel
Barney Taxel & Co.
216/431-2400

Recipe Credits

Oat Bran & Apple Waffle with Apricots, see page 160
Servings: Yields 12 waffles

profiles by reducing both total cholesterol and LDL levels. If you are very overweight (more than 20% over your desired weight, as given in the table in the appendix), gradual weight loss will probably bring down your cholesterol level. Even if you have only 10, 15, or 20 pounds to lose, a well-balanced weight reduction program can help to lower your blood cholesterol significantly. If your blood pressure is above normal, weight loss may help to correct this problem as well. Attaining and maintaining a healthy weight can be the ultimate boon to your cardiovascular system and to your overall health.

DIET MADE EASY

If you are overweight, it probably took many months, even years, for your body to have gotten into the shape that it is in now. You need to accept the fact that it will take time for you to reverse the process, to get into good physical shape, to become fit and healthy. By committing yourself to a well-balanced weight loss plan, you will be able to:

- lose weight gradually, safely, permanently
- enjoy a wide variety of foods in moderate amounts
- lower high blood pressure
- reduce elevated blood cholesterol
- increase both the length of your life and your physical and emotional health

A well-balanced diet that supplies your body with the proper amounts of nutrients does not have to be a confusing maze of dietary unknowns, nor need it be like a prison sentence that destroys your culinary pleasures. This book provides you with the U.S. Department of Agriculture's food values that will enable you to build a diet based on a wide variety of foods. Also included are "A Month Of Menus" with nutritious and delicious low-calorie meals and snack ideas (that are low in cholesterol, saturated fats and sodium).

THE PHYSIOLOGY OF NUTRITION

Unless the reader understands the basic physiology of nutrition, he or she will be unable to make an informed judgment about dietary management programs.

Carbohydrates come in two forms: simple carbohydrates, such as sugar, and complex carbohydrates (fruits, vegetables, and grains). All carbohydrates consist of combinations of fructose and/or glucose molecules. Simple carbohydrates (candy, for instance) are rapidly absorbed into the bloodstream, causing a brisk rise in blood sugar. This rapid rise is often followed by a dip in the blood sugar level, causing the feeling of hunger.

The complex carbohydrates take a longer time to break down into simple sugars and therefore enter the blood stream at a slower rate with less impact on the blood glucose than simple sugars.

Proteins are the building blocks of all the organs and muscles in the body and are complex molecules made up of long chains of amino acids. Dietary proteins must be broken down to their amino acid constituents by enzymes before they can enter the blood stream. Amino acids are essential raw materials needed for the repair, maintenance, and growth of body tissues. Excess amino acids can be converted into glucose for fuel or converted into fat for storage. Nitrogen waste products produced by these conversions are excreted by healthy kidneys. If there is renal disease or insufficiency, the buildup of nitrogen in the blood from protein metabolism may cause a serious medical condition called uremia.

Fat is essential for normal metabolism and your health. Fat

plays an important role insulating tissues, thereby providing internal temperature control and support the internal organs of the body. Fat is the storage form of energy required for muscular work.

Fat is a dietary essential because it transports certain vitamins (the "fat-soluble" vitamins A, D, E, and K) as well as the essential fatty acids required for growth and health. Fat also provides flavor and satiety, increasing eating enjoyment.

It would be undesirable and practically impossible — to eliminate all fat from your diet. The key to a prudent diet is to moderate total fat intake and to emphasize the more healthful types of fat.

Before making a serious commitment to a weight reduction diet and exercise program, you should have a complete medical exam by your physician. Losing pounds is just the beginning. Be prepared to follow an intelligent approach to nutrition and physical activity that will remain with you for the rest of your life. In the beginning, you will feel satisfaction as your weight declines. If you relapse, you may feel anguish and depression. Be prepared for these mixed emotions. Conquering your obesity and lowering your risk for all the possible medical and surgical events that are associated with it will raise your self esteem and bring about a "good feeling" that you may not have had for years. There will be no more self-pity, resentment, or guilt feelings in regard to food. If you are diabetic you will find it much easier to control your blood sugar. If you have Type II (adult-onset) diabetes it may even return to normal.

The obese person must accept an intelligent, nutritious diet plan, adopt a daily exercise routine, and remain on this regimen for the rest of his life. Your health and your appearance will make it all worthwhile.

The First Magic Key: Listen to Your Body

Learn to listen to your body. Do not eat automatically, simply because it is mealtime. Your body knows when it requires food. You need not go hungry. Make whole grains, vegetables and fruits the staples of your diet. By cutting fatty foods from your diet and replacing them with low-calorie food stuffs that are naturally more filling, you will automatically reduce your caloric intake painlessly. Gradually, healthful diet habits can replace a lifelong pattern of binge eating and dieting. Your new diet will eventually become permanent, natural and enjoyable. Normal hunger is the body's signal to eat. Satiation with nutritious filling foods is magic key number one. While consuming less calories, you need never go hungry.

The Second Magic Key: Exercise

As noted, weight control is based on a simple caloric equation: take in more calories than you use up in day-to-day activity and you gain weight; take in less calories than your body is using and you will lose weight. However, a low-calorie diet without regular exercise can gradually lose effectiveness, as the body requires fewer calories as pounds shed. This is one of the major reasons why over 90 percent of all dieters fail. They grow discouraged or depressed with slowed success because they cut calories without adding exercise. Exercise is the key to long-term weight loss success!

This does not mean you need to transform yourself into a marathon runner or professional athlete. In order to enhance the weight loss process, you need only begin a regular program of "aerobic" exercise such as walking, jogging, bicycling, or swimming. By exercising 20-30 minutes 3-4 times a week, you will burn off extra calories and tone your muscles. Plus, regular exercise will help reduce your blood pressure and improve your blood lipid profile by lowering total cholesterol and boosting your HDL level. Aerobic exercise strengthens the cardiovascular system and speeds up the rate of weight loss — a double plus!

Slow and Easy

In order to be successful in your weight-loss efforts, it is essential for you to be patient. Begin your new low-cholesterol, low-sodium, low-calorie diet slowly and carefully. Use the sample menus provided to ease your palate and your psyche into the healthful way of eating. Begin on your exercise program in this same manner; that is, slowly and carefully. If you overdo with physical activity, you will probably become stiff, sore, and turned off to exercise. Start with a daily walk around the block, and advance gradually from there. Remember, it has taken some time for your body to get into its current shape. Accordingly, it will take some time for you to diet and exercise yourself into the fit new you. Go for it!

MINERALS

Minerals are naturally occurring elements, of which seventeen are essential to human health. These "essential" minerals are required to form healthy body tissues and regulate various vital body functions. Several of them play important roles in cardiovascular function and health.

Calcium is essential for bone formation and strength, and assists in nerve transmission, muscle contraction, and heartbeat. Inadequate intake of calcium has been associated with high blood pressure and osteoporosis. Women over age 50 should take at least 1500mg/day. Men over age 65 need 1000mg/day. One Tums® tablet contains 500mg.

Foods rich in calcium include:
- skim milk
- non-fat yogurt
- low-fat and non-fat cheeses

- salmon and sardines (with bones)
- green leafy vegetables (broccoli, spinach)
- tofu

Magnesium is essential for many major metabolic processes. It plays an important role in the functioning of nerves and muscles, including the heart. Along with calcium and phosphorus, it is one of the "bone minerals." Deficiencies can occur with alcoholism, diuretic ("water pill") use, and inadequate dietary intake. A diet deficient in this mineral may lead to high blood pressure, heart disease or strokes. "Hard" water contains calcium and magnesium. Those who drink "hard" water have a lower incidence of cardiovascular disease.

Foods rich in magnesium include:
- fresh green vegetables
- oil rich seeds and nuts (especially almonds)
- dried beans and peas
- nuts
- whole grains, including oats
- seafood
- tofu (soybean curd)

Potassium is critical for regulating water balance and proper heartbeat rhythm as well as many other vital cellular functions. Gradual potassium depletion can occur with heavy sweating, diarrhea, and certain diuretics. Diets deficient in this essential mineral have been associated with high blood pressure.

Potassium-rich foods include:
- citrus fruits and juices
- bananas, strawberries, dried fruits
- tomatoes, broccoli, brussel sprouts, carrots, spinach
- corn, potatoes, sweet potatoes
- skim milk

Sodium and Your Health

Sodium is an essential mineral for life that plays an important role as a major constituent in body fluids. It is an abundant mineral found virtually in all foods (ordinary salt). It is essential for proper nerve transmission and muscle contraction. A depletion of this mineral can occur with dehydration due to illness, diuretic use, or heavy sweating. However, sodium is so ample in the typical diet that it is easy to obtain adequate amounts. In fact, most Americans consume far too much sodium. Too high a sodium intake tends to cause water retention, increasing blood volume and causing high blood pressure in susceptible individuals. For those individuals who are "sodium sensitive," it is imperative to restrict sodium intake. The medical community (including the U. S. Surgeon General) suggest that everyone, particularly those over age 45, moderate sodium intake. For many people with hypertension, adherence to a low-sodium diet can dramatically lower high blood pressure. The simplest way to reduce the sodium in your diet is by not using the salt shaker (salt is "sodium chloride," containing 40 percent sodium or 2,000mg per teaspoon); avoid or minimize your intake of foods from the High Sodium Foods List that follows. Reduce your sodium intake to a prudent, healthful level. Salt substitutes contain potassium chloride and may be used on low-sodium diets. Cooking changes the flavor of these products, therefore, they should be used only as a condiment at the table. Low-salt products contain much less sodium than regular salt, but they still have too much for regular use on a sodium-restricted diet.

High Sodium Foods List

bacon	caviar
biscuits	chips
bouillon	chipped beef
canned fish	cold cuts
canned meats	convenience foods

corned beef
crackers
  (unless unsalted)
dips
dried meats
fast foods
frozen dinners
ham
ketchup
lox
medications: antacids,
  antibiotics, buffered
  headache remedies,
  cough medicines,
  laxatives,
  sedatives, sodium
  bicarbonate
  (baking soda), certain
  mouthwashes
packaged dinners, mixes
pastrami

pickles
pretzels
relishes
salts: celery, garlic, onion,
  sea, seasoned, table,
  monosodium glutamate
  (MSG)
sauerkraut
sausages
seasonings: cooking wines,
  meat extracts, meat
  tenderizers and mari-
  nades
smoked fish
smoked meats
soups
soysauce
stews
tomato juice
vegetable juice cocktail

FIBER

Fiber is the indigestible residue of food that is not absorbed from the intestinal tract. Fiber has long been recognized as an important food element that plays a major role in the digestive process. Since fiber is largely indigestible, fibrous foods pass rapidly through the digestive tract, assisting in efficient elimination and preventing constipation, hemorrhoids, and other bowel disorders.

There are several types of fiber, each with different physical properties and health roles. The "insoluble" fiber — so-called roughage — is the type found in wheat bran, whole wheat products, fruits and vegetables. It speeds digestion, but does not lower cholesterol. The "soluble" fiber is water soluble and is found in fruits, vegetables, oat bran, dried beans and peas. This type of fiber serves an essential function by interfering with the absorption of fats and cholesterol, therefore diets rich in soluble fiber can help to lower blood lipid levels. Most complex carbohydrates are mixtures of soluble and insoluble fibers.

It is not possible to judge the soluble fiber content from the appearance of the food. High soluble fiber foods are not necessarily course, crunchy or stringy. Cooking fruits and vegetables destroys much of the fiber.

Most Americans consume inadequate amounts of dietary fiber. A prudent diet includes ample servings of foods rich in "complex carbohydrates" (starches) and fiber, emphasizing the dietary sources of soluble fibers:

Grains: oat bran, oat bran cereals, breads, muffins

Fruit: especially apples, berries, grapes, peaches, plums, and dried fruit

Vegetables: especially sweet potatoes, asparagus, spinach, cucumbers, broccoli, brussel sprouts, cabbage, carrots, cauliflower, corn, beans and peas, greens, and potatoes (with skin)

ENERGY EXPENDITURE BY A 150 POUND PERSON IN VARIOUS ACTIVITIES**

Choose from the following physical activities to burn calories while getting fit. Aerobic exercises are indicated by an asterisk (*).

Activity Energy Cost: Calories per Hour

Rest and Light Activity 50-200
Lying down or sleeping 80
Sitting 100
Driving an automobile 120
Standing 140
Domestic work 180

Moderate Activity 200-350
*Bicycling(5mph) 210
*Walking (2mph) 210
Gardening 220
Gymnastics 220
Canoeing (2mph) 230
Golf. 250
Lawn mowing (power mower).......................... 250
Bowling 270
*Lawn mowing (hand mower) 270
Fencing 300
Rowboating (2mph) 300
*Walking (4mph) 300
Badminton 300
Horseback riding (trotting) 350
*Square dancing 350
Volleyball 350
*Roller skating.. 350

Vigorous Activity .... over 350
Table tennis 360
Ditch digging (hand shovel) 400
*Ice skating (10mph) 400
*Skiing, cross country 400
Wood chopping or sawing 400

*Swimming -side stroke 400
    -competitive 520
Tennis 420
*Jogging -12 min/mile 455
    -9 min/mile 645
    -8 min/mile 715
Basketball 460
Water skiing 480
*Hill climbing (100 ft/hour) 490
Skiing, downhill (10mph) 600
Squash and handball 600
*Cycling (13mph) 660
Racquetball 715
*Running -7 min/mile 800
    -6 min/mile 900
*Scull rowing, competitive 840

**Adapted from: U.S. Government Printing Office brochure #040-000-0037-1 ("Exercise and Weight Control"). Where available, actual measured values have been used, for other values a "best guess" was made.

IMPORTANT NOTES:

* Frozen or canned fruits should be packed in their own juices — without added sugar or syrup.
* Vegetables should be fresh or frozen without added salt or sauces; low-sodium canned are acceptable alternatives.
* Breads and cereals should be whole grain products.
* Whole-grain pastas and brown rice are preferred.
* Crackers and breadsticks should be whole grain and *unsalted*.
* Prepare popcorn without added oil, butter, or salt by using hot-air popper or oil-free microwave popcorn.
* Prepare dried beans and peas by soaking overnight in cold water before cooking; read labels on canned beans to check for (and avoid) added salt and fats.

* Peanut butter should be old-fashioned or natural brands made without added hydrogenated fats or salt; nuts should be *unsalted*.
* Fish should be prepared by baking, boiling, broiling, or poaching; brush with olive oil (lightly) and season with herbs, if desired.
* Canned fish should be low-sodium when possible.
* Poultry should be skinless and prepared by baking, boiling, broiling, or roasting; dark meat is significantly lower in fat than white meat.
* Meats should be lean, well-trimmed, and prepared by baking, boiling, broiling, or roasting; use small amounts of lean cuts to *complement* the meal, rather than serving meat as the main dish.
* Limit egg intake to 1-2 yolks weekly; use egg whites to stretch recipes (1 whole egg + 2 eggwhites for 2 whole eggs) or use egg substitutes (read labels to ensure products are no-cholesterol and low-sodium choices).
* Select skim or low-fat (1%) milk, non-fat or low-fat yogurt and uncreamed, or low-fat (1% or 2%) cottage cheese.
* Select low-fat or non-fat cheeses (less than 3 grams fat/oz) by reading labels' use *light* dustings of grated Parmesan cheese to add flavor (and nutrition) to vegetables and casserole-type dishes.
* Use *small* amounts of olive oil with vinegar and lemon to dress salads, or choose olive oil-based salad dressings-and use *sparingly*; low-calorie, low-fat, and fat-free salad dressings are preferred.

DINING OUT DO'S AND DON'TS

Just because you are being careful in your food selections, you do not have to give up restaurants altogether, nor opt for brown bag lunches every day. By following a few basic rules, you can make wise food choices almost anywhere—

whether at a fast food outlet, a gourmet banquet or a local cafeteria. In order to make menu selections that are low in saturated fat, cholesterol, sodium, and calories, keep in mind the following:

DO'S	DON'TS
Appetizers:	
fresh vegetables,	bouillons or consommes
fresh fruits,	soups or chowders,
fruit salad, unsweetened,	marinated vegetables,
fresh fruit juice,	salted crackers,
seafood, steamed or cocktails	chips, dips, nuts, caviar
Salads:	
green, tossed	mayonnaise-based salads,
chef's with poultry,	potato salad, egg salad,
low-calorie dressings,	creamy coleslaw,
oil and vinegar,	chef's with egg, fatty
	meats,
Note: Request that dressings	spinach with egg and
be served on the side	bacon,
be served on the side	commercial salad
Vegetables:	
any plain, fresh	buttered,canned, creamed,
	fried, marinated,pickled,
	seasoned, sauced
Breads:	
whole grain breads,	garlic bread,
breadsticks, unsalted,	egg or cheese breads,
French or Italian,	hard rolls,
pita bread,	submarine rolls,

crackers, unsalted,
dinner rolls, plain,
English muffins,
bagels

breadsticks, salted,
crackers, butter or cheese,
crackers, salted,
biscuits, croissants,
muffins, butter rolls,
sweet rolls

Meat:
lean, trimmed cuts, baked,
boiles, broiled, raosted
no gravies or sauces

breaded, fried, marinated
cuts, gravies, stews,
sauces

Poultry:
chicken or turkey,
baked, boiled,
broiled, roasted,
no gravies or sauces

goose, duck, skin
removed, breaded,
fried, marinated cuts,
gravies, stews, sauces
(cream, cheese, soy,
tomato, white)

Fish and Shellfish:
any (prepared with minimal
use of margarine—baked,
boiled, broiled, poached

breaded, fried,
frozen fillets,
dried, pickled, smoked

Desserts:
angel food cake,
frozen fruit juices,
sorbets, fruits--fresh,
baked, dried, poached

rich sweets: cake, candy,
cookies, doughnuts, ice
cream, pastries, puddings

Beverages:

fruit juices,
skim, low-fat milk,
coffee, tea,
light beers, dry
wines

tomato juice,
vegetable juice,
cocktails,
shakes, eggnog cream,
cream substitutes,
sweetened alcoholic,
beverages and liqueurs

Extras:

lemon juice, herbs
spices
cottage cheese, low-fat

pickles, relishes
mustard, ketchup,
cocktail sauce,
steak sauce,
Worcestershire sauce,
mayonnaise, sour cream,
bacon bits

ADDITIONAL NOTE:

Read menus carefully to avoid selections described as the following:

- buttered, butter, butter sauce
- creamed, creamy, cream sauce
- fried, french fried, pan fried, crispy
- au gratin, cheese sauce, escalloped
- a la king, bernaise, hollandaise
- casserole, hash, pot pie, stew
- marinated, pickled, sauteed, smoked
- all you can eat

Remember, the key to successful dining out is to follow a low-fat diet plan. When this is impossible, choose your foods carefully and eat them in moderation. It may prove wiser not to do, than to overdo!

DESIRED WEIGHTS

HOW MUCH SHOULD YOU WEIGH?

Normal weights for Americans as determined by the Metropolitan Life Insurance Co., based on small, medium or large frames:

Hgt.	Weights for Men			Weights for Women		
	Small	Medium	Large	Small	Medium	Large
4-10				102-111	109-121	118-131
4-11				103-113	111-123	120-134
5-0				104-115	113-126	122-137
5-1				106-118	115-129	125-140
5-2	128-134	131-141	138-150	108-121	118-132	128-143
5-3	130-136	133-143	140-153	111-124	121-135	131-147
5-4	132-138	135-145	142-156	114-127	124-138	134-151
5-5	134-140	137-148	144-160	117-130	127-141	137-155
5-6	136-142	139-151	146-164	120-133	130-144	140-159
5-7	138-145	142-154	149-168	123-136	133-147	143-163
5-8	140-148	145-157	152-172	126-139	136-150	146-167
5-9	142-151	148-160	155-176	129-142	139-153	149-170
5-10	144-154	151-163	158-180	132-145	142-156	152-173
5-11	146-157	154-166	161-184	135-148	145-159	155-176
6-0	149-160	157-170	164-188	138-151	148-162	158-179
6-1	152-164	160-174	168-192			
6-2	155-168	164-178	172-197			
6-3	158-172	167-182	176-202			
6-4	162-176	171-187	181-207			

Weight in Pounds according to frame (in indoor clothing weighing 5 lbs. for men, and 3 lbs. for women: shoes with 1" heels).

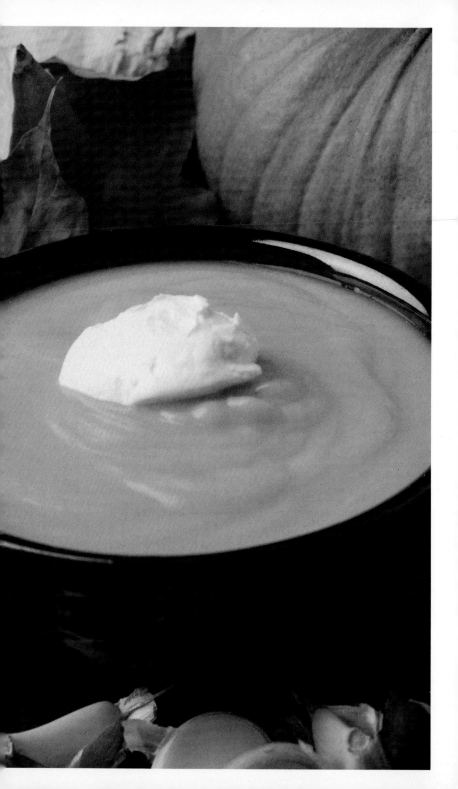

Pumpkin-Cumin Soup
Rich in flavor and low in fat! This recipe is a "souper" start to any meal.

Photo Credits
Photography by Barney Taxel
Barney Taxel & Co.
216/431-2400

Recipe Credits
Pumpkin-Cumin Soup, see page 52
Servings: 6

2
Appetizers

Low Fat Humus Dip

> **SERVES 4**
>
> **Dip: 1 16-ounce can garbanzo beans**
> **1 teaspoon sesame tahini**
> **1 teaspoon extra-virgin olive oil**
> **1 teaspoon chopped fresh garlic**
> **1 tablespoon water**
> **1/4 teaspoon black pepper**
> **2 teaspoons fresh lemon juice**
> **1/8 teaspoon cayenne (red) pepper (or to taste)**
> **1/2 teaspoon cumin**
> **1/8 teaspoon salt (optional)**
>
> **Topping: 2 hard-boiled eggs, yolks removed**
> **2 tablespoons chopped black olives**
> **1 sprig fresh parsley or other greens**

1. *Rinse and drain garbanzo beans. Discard outer coverings.*
2. *Combine all dip ingredients with garbanzo beans.*
3. *Process in a blender until smooth. Place in a serving dish.*
4. *For topping: remove and discard yolks from boiled eggs; chop whites into small pieces; mix with olives.*
5. *Sprinkle topping over dip. Top with parsley.*
6. *Serve with pita bread or raw vegetables.*

☑ *Nutrition Information*

Calories	152
Carbohydrates (grams)	20
Proteins (grams)	8
Cholesterol (milligrams)	53
Sodium (milligrams)	135
Fat (grams)	5
Saturated Fat (grams)	1

Ratatouille

SERVES 6
1 large red onion, chopped
2 medium-size green peppers, chopped
1 clove garlic, minced
3 medium-size ripe tomatoes, peeled, seeded, and diced
1 small eggplant, diced
1 small zucchini, diced
1/4 cup tomato puree
1 tablespoon freshly chopped parsley
1/2 teaspoon whole oregano
1/4 teaspoon crushed peppercorns
1 tablespoon freshly grated Parmesan cheese

1. *In a Dutch oven, steam onion, green pepper and garlic with 1/4 cup water or chicken broth.*
2. *Add tomatoes, eggplant, zucchini, tomato puree and seasonings.*
3. *Stir thoroughly.*
4. *Cover and bake at 375 for 20 minutes.*
5. *Uncover, sprinkle with cheese and bake 20 minutes more.*

☑ *Nutrition Information*

Calories	55
Carbohydrates (grams)	11.6
Proteins (grams)	2.1
Cholesterol (milligrams)	0
Sodium (milligrams)	71
Fat (grams)	0.7
Saturated Fat (grams)	0

Apple-Stuffed Mushroom Caps

YIELDS 32 MUSHROOMS
32 large fresh mushrooms
Vegetable cooking spray
3 tablespoons finely chopped celery
1/2 cup minced apple
2 tablespoons finely chopped walnuts, toasted
2 tablespoons fine, dry breadcrumbs
1 tablespoon chopped fresh parsley
1 tablespoon crumbled blue cheese
2 teaspoons lemon juice

1. *Clean mushrooms and remove stems.*
2. *Finely chop 1/3 cup stems; reserve remaining stems.*
3. *Heat a nonstick skillet coated with cooking spray over medium-high heat.*
4. *When hot add reserved mushroom stems and celery; saute until tender.*
5. *In a bowl combine celery mixture, apple and next 5 ingredients.*
6. *Fill each mushroom cap with 1-1/2 teaspoons mixture.*
7. *Bake in a casserole dish at 350 for 15 minutes.*

☑ *Nutrition Information*

Calories	13
Carbohydrates (grams)	1.9
Proteins (grams)	0.7
Cholesterol (milligrams)	0
Sodium (milligrams)	8
Fat (grams)	0.5
Saturated Fat (grams)	0

Minted Millet, Cucumber and Garbanzo Salad

SERVES 6
Lemon-mint dressing: 3 tablespoons olive oil
1/3 cup lemon juice
1 cup fresh mint leaves, loosely packed
1/2 cup chopped parsley

Salad: 2-3 Kirby cucumbers, diced
1 medium to large red onion, diced
16 to 20 ounces can garbanzo beans
1 cup uncooked millet
2 teaspoons olive oil
1/4 teaspoon ground cinnamon
1/4 teaspoon ground cardamom
2-1/2 cup boiling water
1 strip lemon peel

1. In a large bowl combine all dressing ingredients; mix well.
2. Add cucumbers, garbanzo beans and onions to dressing; marinate 30 minutes.
3. Rinse millet and drain through a fine strainer.
4. Cook over medium-low heat, stirring frequently, for 10 minutes or until water evaporates.
5. Drizzle millet with oil and stir in spices.
6. Add boiling water and reduce heat to a low simmer.
7. Add lemon peel, cover and simmer 25 minutes or until all water is absorbed.
8. Remove lemon peel; fluff millet and allow to cool.
9. Combine millet with vegetables and dressing; mix well.

☑ **Nutrition Information**

Calories	324
Carbohydrates (grams)	46
Proteins (grams)	15.5
Cholesterol (milligrams)	2
Sodium (milligrams)	7.2
Fat (grams)	11.3
Saturated Fat (grams)	2.2

Basmati and Wild Rice with Tangerines and Pine Nuts

SERVES 6
1 cup wild rice
7 cups water (3 cups and 4 cups separately
1/2 cup Basmati rice, rinsed and drained
3/4 cup fresh tangerine juice, about 4 tangerines
1/2 cup dried currants
3 tangerines
Champagne vinegar
2 teaspoon light olive oil
2 tablespoon pine nuts, toasted

1. Place rice in a large saucepan; cover with 1 quart water and boil.
2. Reduce heat to a gentle boil; cover and cook about 35 minutes (grains should be tender but chewy).
3. Bring remaining 3 cups water to a boil in a separate pan; add basmati rice.
4. Cook 8-10 minutes; drain and cool; then add to wild rice.
5. Heat tangerine juice over medium heat just until boiling.
6. Pour juice over currants.
7. Peel and section tangerines; remove seeds and threads.
8. Toss rice with currants, tangerine juice, 1/2 tablespoon champagne vinegar, olive oil.
9. Add tangerines and pine nuts just before serving at room temperature.

☑ Nutrition Information

Calories	238
Carbohydrates (grams)	47
Proteins (grams)	7.1
Cholesterol (milligrams)	0
Sodium (milligrams)	5
Fat (grams)	3.6
Saturated Fat (grams)	0.4

Couscous Salad with Apricots, Pine Nuts and Ginger

SERVES 4
1 cup couscous - uncooked
1/2 cup water
1 cup fresh orange juice
2 tablespoons olive oil
Champagne vinegar
8 dried apricots, thinly sliced, about 1/3 cup
1 tablespoon dried currants
1 tablespoon golden raisins
2 teaspoons grated fresh ginger
1/4 medium-size red onion, finely diced, about 1/2 cup
2 tablespoons pine nuts, toasted

1. *Pour couscous into a bowl; set aside.*
2. *In a saucepan, combine water, orange juice, olive oil and 2 tablespoons vinegar.*
3. *Bring just to a boil.*
4. *Stir in dried fruit and ginger.*
5. *Pour over couscous.*
6. *Cover and let stand 20 minutes.*
7. *Boil a small pot of water. Drop in onion for 15 seconds; drain.*
8. *Toss onion with a few splashes of vinegar.*
9. *When couscous is done fluff it with a fork.*
10. *Toss with pine nuts and onion.*
11. *Add a splash of vinegar and serve.*

Nutrition Information

Calories	365
Carbohydrates (grams)	62
Proteins (grams)	9
Cholesterol (milligrams)	0
Sodium (milligrams)	9
Fat (grams)	10
Saturated Fat (grams)	1.2

Pumpkin-Cumin Soup

SERVES 6
Vegetable cooking spray
1 tablespoon diet margarine
1 cup chopped onion
2 (10-1/2 ounce) cans low sodium chicken broth,
undiluted and divided
2 tablespoons all purpose flour
1 (16-ounce) can cooked, mashed pumpkin
1-1/2 teaspoon ground cumin
1 cup skim milk
1/2 cup plain nonfat yogurt

1. In a large nonstick skillet coated with cooking spray, melt diet margarine over medium heat.
2. Add onion and saute until tender.
3. Stir in 1 can chicken broth.
4. Boil; cover and reduce heat; simmer 15 minutes.
5. Place mixture in a blender; add flour and process until smooth.
6. Return mixture to pan add remaining chicken broth, pumpkin and cumin.
7. Boil then reduce heat; cover and simmer 10 minutes.
8. Stir in milk and cook until heated through (do not boil).
9. Ladle soup into individual bowls and top with 1 tablespoon yogurt.

✓ Nutrition Information

Calories	90
Carbohydrates (grams)	15
Proteins (grams)	5
Cholesterol (milligrams)	1.2
Sodium (milligrams)	93
Fat (grams)	1.6
Saturated Fat (grams)	0.3

Lemon-Dijon Marinated Shrimp

YIELDS 36 shrimps
1 quart water
36 unpeeled medium shrimp (1-1/2 pounds)
1 cup water
1/3 cup lemon juice
2 tablespoons Dijon mustard
2 cloves garlic, minced
3/4 teaspoon dried whole dillweed
1/2 teaspoon peeled, minced gingerroot
1/4 teaspoon crushed red pepper
36 fresh snow pea pods, trimmed

1. Boil 1 quart of water; add shrimp and cook 3-5 minutes.
2. Drain shrimp and rinse; chill.
3. Peel and clean shrimp; place in a baking dish; set aside.
4. In a small bowl combine 1 cup water and next 6 ingredients; stir well.
5. Pour over shrimp and toss.
6. Cover and refrigerate 5 hours .
7. Steam snow peas over boiling water 3-5 minutes; remove from steamer and chill.
8. Wrap each shrimp in a snow pea and secure with a toothpick.

☑ Nutrition Information

Calories	13
Carbohydrates (grams)	0.6
Proteins (grams)	2.1
Cholesterol (milligrams)	18
Sodium (milligrams)	46
Fat (grams)	0.2
Saturated Fat (grams)	0

Marinated Mozzarella Appetizer

YIELDS 32 SERVINGS
8 ounces nonfat mozzarella cheese, diced
1 (7 ounce) jar roasted red peppers in water, drained
and coarsely   chopped
2 tablespoons minced oregano
1/2 teaspoon freshly ground pepper
1-1/2 tablespoon lemon juice
2 teaspoon olive oil
16 each, endive and radicchio leaves

1. *Combine first 6 ingredients in a bowl and stir well.*
2. *Cover and chill 6 hours.*
3. *Spoon 1 tablespoon cheese mixture onto each lettuce leaf.*
4. *Arrange on a serving platter, cover and chill 2 hours before serving.*

☑ *Nutrition Information*

Calories	23
Carbohydrates (grams)	0.8
Proteins (grams)	1.9
Cholesterol (milligrams)	4
Sodium (milligrams)	108
Fat (grams)	1.4
Saturated Fat (grams)	0.8

Eastern European Sweet and Sour Meatballs

YIELDS 32 MEATBALLS
1-1/2 pounds ground turkey
1 cup plain breadcrumbs
1 cup egg substitute
1 4-6 ounce can tomato paste and 1 can water
1 16 ounce can whole tomatoes
Juice of 2 lemons
3/4 cup sugar
1 diced onion
1 15 ounce can wholeberry cranberry sauce
3/4 cup raisins

---

1. Mix ground turkey, breadcrumbs and egg substitute.
2. Roll into 32-1 inch meatballs; set aside.
3. Mix together tomato paste, tomatoes and next 5 ingredients in a large pot.
4. Heat thoroughly.
5. Add meatballs and boil.
6. Reduce heat and cover; simmer 1 hour stirring frequently.

☑ **Nutrition Information**

Calories	107
Carbohydrates (grams)	18
Proteins (grams)	4.5
Cholesterol (milligrams)	6.7
Sodium (milligrams)	185
Fat (grams)	1.9
Saturated Fat (grams)	0.5

Roast Garlic Pate Toasts

YIELDS 32 SERVINGS
2 large heads garlic
Olive-oil flavored cooking spray
8 sundried tomatoes (not packed in oil)
boiling water
1/2 cup nonfat cottage cheese
3 ounces goat cheese
1 tablespoon Dijon mustard
2 tablespoons minced fresh basil
32 Melba crackers

1. *In a small bowl cover tomatoes with boiling water; let stand 10 minutes. Drain and reserve tomatoes.*
2. *Remove skin from garlic, leaving cloves intact.*
3. *Cut a thin slice from the top of each bulb of garlic to expose the cloves. Coat tops of garlic with cooking spray.*
4. *Place garlic, cut side up, on a piece of aluminum foil.*
5. *Sprinkle 1 tablespoon water on garlic. Fold up aluminum foil over garlic, sealing tightly.*
6. *Bake garlic at 350 for 1 hour; remove from oven and place in refrigerator to chill for 1 hour.*
7. *Squeeze garlic cloves to remove pulp; place in a blender.*
8. *Add cottage cheese and mustard to blender and process until smooth.*
9. *Pat tomatoes dry and chop finely.*
10. *Stir tomatoes and basil into garlic mixture.*
11. *Serve chilled or at room temperature with melba crackers.*

☑ Nutrition Information

Calories	29
Carbohydrates (grams)	3.3
Proteins (grams)	2.1
Cholesterol (milligrams)	2.8
Sodium (milligrams)	124
Fat (grams)	0.7
Saturated Fat (grams)	0.5

Orange and Olive Salad

SERVES 4
4 ounces unsweetened orange juice
3 cups orange segments, packed in their own juice
20 small black olives, sliced

1. *Mix oranges and orange juice.*
2. *Spoon onto 4 individual serving plates.*
3. *Top with sliced olives.*

☑ <u>*Nutrition Information*</u>

Calories	102
Carbohydrates (grams)	20
Proteins (grams)	1.9
Cholesterol (milligrams)	0
Sodium (milligrams)	96
Fat (grams)	3.5
Saturated Fat (grams)	0.3

Shrimp and Crabmeat Canapes

SERVES 72
3 cups water
1 teaspoon liquid shrimp and crab boil seasoning
1 pound unpeeled small fresh shrimp
1/2 pound fresh lump crab meat, drained
1 cup finely chopped celery
1/3 cup soft bread crumbs
1/3 cup non-fat mayonnaise
1/4 cup plain non-fat yogurt
1 tablespoon chopped pimento
1 teaspoon lemon juice
3/4 teaspoon low sodium Worcestershire sauce
1/8 teaspoon dry mustard
1/8 teaspoon ground red pepper
72 melba rounds

1. Boil water and seasoning in a saucepan; add shrimp and cook 3-5 minutes.
2. Drain shrimp; rinse and chill.
3. Peel and clean shrimp; chop shrimp.
4. Mix together shrimp, crab meat and remaining ingredients, except melba rounds.
5. Top each melba round with 2 teaspoons shrimp mixture.

☑ *Nutrition Information*

Calories	30
Carbohydrates (grams)	4
Proteins (grams)	2.2
Cholesterol (milligrams)	11
Sodium (milligrams)	75
Fat (grams)	0.2
Saturated Fat (grams)	0

3
Entrees

Paella

SERVES 4

2 pounds meaty chicken pieces
1/8 teaspoon pepper
1 tablespoon olive oil
2 cups chicken broth
1 cup long grain rice
1 medium onion, cut into thin wedges
1/2 cup chopped celery
1 2-ounce jar sliced pimiento
2 cloves garlic, minced
1/2 teaspoon dried oregano, crushed
1/8 teaspoon powdered saffron
1 9-ounce package frozen artichoke hearts
4 ounces fresh or frozen shelled shrimp
8 small fresh clams or mussels in shells, washed

1. *Skin chicken and rinse; pat dry. Season chicken with pepper.*
2. *Heat oil in a Dutch oven; cook chicken pieces, uncovered, for 10-15 minutes.*
3. *Turn chicken pieces to brown evenly; remove from Dutch oven.*
4. *In Dutch oven combine chicken broth, uncooked rice, celery, onion, pimento, garlic and spices.*
5. *Add cooked chicken and bring to a boil.*
6. *Reduce heat to low and simmer, covered for 15 minutes.*
7. *Add artichokes and seafood to pan; cover and cook 10-15 minutes more.*

☑ Nutrition Information

Calories	432
Carbohydrates (grams)	47
Proteins (grams)	36
Cholesterol (milligrams)	111
Sodium (milligrams)	670
Fat (grams)	10
Saturated Fat (grams)	2

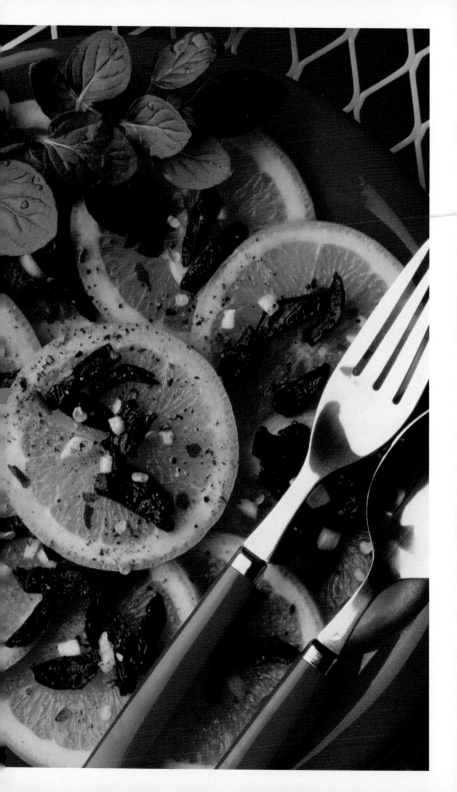

Orange Olive Salad

The tastes of sweet and sharp compliment each other in this simple and nutritious dessert.

Photo Credits
Photography by Barney Taxel
Barney Taxel & Co.
216/431-2400

Recipe Credits
Orange Olive Salad, see page 57
Servings: 4

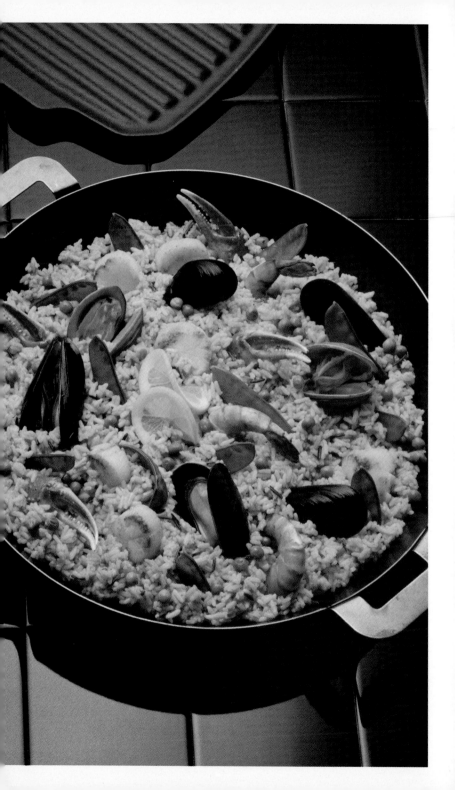

Paella

A heart-healthy tradition from the kitchens of Spain.

Photo Credits
Photography by Barney Taxel
Barney Taxel & Co.
216/431-2400

Recipe Credits
Paella, see page 60
Servings: 4

Chicken Cacciatore

SERVES 4
1 pound skinless, boneless chicken breast
1/8 teaspoon pepper
1 cup sliced mushrooms
1/2 cup sliced onion
1 cup sliced green pepper
2 cup peeled seeded and diced whole tomato
3/4 cup low sodium chicken broth
1 teaspoon whole oregano

1. *Sprinkle chicken breasts with pepper and place in a nonstick skillet.*
2. *Brown over medium heat; remove to plate when done.*
3. *Add vegetables, chicken broth and oregano to skillet; simmer approximately 15 minutes.*
4. *Return chicken to skillet; heat and serve.*

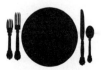

☑ **Nutrition Information**

Calories	144
Carbohydrates (grams)	12
Proteins (grams)	19
Cholesterol (milligrams)	46
Sodium (milligrams)	64
Fat (grams)	2.6
Saturated Fat (grams)	0.6

Pesto-Onion-Pepper Pizza

YIELDS 8 SLICES
1 (14.5 oz.) package focaccia or 1 (1-pound) Italian
cheese-flavored thin pizza crust (such as Boboli)
2 tablespoons pesto basil sauce
2 large garlic cloves, thinly sliced
1/2 cup (2 oz.) preshredded part-skim mozzarella cheese
1/3 cup (1 ounce) preshredded fresh Parmesan cheese
1/2 teaspoon coarsely ground pepper
2 tablespoons thinly sliced fresh basil leaves
1/2 cup sliced onion
1/2 cup sliced green pepper

1. *Preheat oven to 450.*
2. *Place crust on a large pizza stone.*
3. *Spread pesto sauce over crust; spread onion,pepper and garlic over pesto sauce; season with pepper;top with cheeses.*
4. *Bake for 8 minutes.*
5. *Sprinkle with basil and serve.*

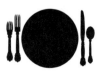

☑ Nutrition Information

Calories	388
Carbohydrates (grams)	56.5
Proteins (grams)	17.9
Cholesterol (milligrams)	14
Sodium (milligrams)	794
Fat (grams)	12.4
Saturated Fat (grams)	5.3

Swordfish Italiano

SERVES 4
1-1/2 pounds swordfish
1/2 teaspoon whole oregano
1 teaspoon paprika
1 tablespoon diet margarine
1 minced garlic clove
1/2 cup chopped green onion (white part only)
1/2 cup chopped celery
1/2 cup chopped green pepper
1/4 cup tomato juice
1 cup peeled and diced, fresh or canned tomatoes

1. *Rinse and dry swordfish; season with oregano and paprika.*
2. *Place fish in a baking pan.*
3. *Over medium heat, saute garlic, green onion, celery and green pepper in diet margarine.*
4. *Add tomato juice and tomatoes; mix well.*
5. *Pour over fish.*
6. *Bake at 350 for 20 minutes.*

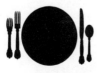

☑ *Nutrition Information*

Calories	260
Carbohydrates (grams)	7
Proteins (grams)	35
Cholesterol (milligrams)	67
Sodium (milligrams)	340
Fat (grams)	9.8
Saturated Fat (grams)	2.3

Tuscan Chicken

SERVES 4
12 medium sized mushrooms
2 tablespoons light margarine
8 skinless chicken thighs
1/4 teaspoon black pepper
1 teaspoon minced garlic
1/2 teaspoon dried rosemary
1 cup dry white wine
1 tablespoon tomato paste
2 small tomatoes; cut into 3/4 inch chunks

1. *In a nonstick skillet brown mushrooms in 1 tablespoon diet margarine; remove to plate.*
2. *Season chicken with pepper; brown 3 minutes each side in remaining diet margarine.*
3. *Reduce heat to low and add garlic and rosemary to skillet; turn chicken and mix well.*
4. *Remove chicken and drippings to plate (do not combine with mushrooms).*
5. *Add wine and tomato paste to skillet and boil down to 1/2 cup; return chicken to skillet.*
6. *Cover and cook over low heat about 20 minutes, turning once.*
7. *Add mushrooms and tomato; heat 2-3 minutes and serve.*

☑ *Nutrition Information*

Calories	293
Carbohydrates (grams)	5
Proteins (grams)	27
Cholesterol (milligrams)	93
Sodium (milligrams)	193
Fat (grams)	14
Saturated Fat (grams)	3.5

Lemon Chicken with Honey Nut Glaze

SERVES 4
1-1/2 pounds of boneless, skinless chicken breast
1/2 teaspoon ground pepper
6 tablespoon fresh lemon juice
2 tablespoon olive oil
Glaze:
1 tablespoon light margarine
2 tablespoon finely chopped walnuts
1/2 cup mild honey

---

1. *In a jar combine pepper, lemon juice and oil; shake to mix.*
2. *Pour mixture over chicken and let stand 20 minutes.*
3. *In a nonstick skillet over medium heat, toast walnuts in diet margarine.*
4. *Add honey; mix and set aside.*
5. *Broil chicken approximately 6 minutes each side; remove to serving dish.*
6. *If necessary reheat glaze; spoon over chicken and serve.*

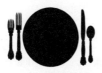

☑ *Nutrition Information*

Calories	360
Carbohydrates (grams)	35
Proteins (grams)	26
Cholesterol (milligrams)	69
Sodium (milligrams)	94
Fat (grams)	13
Saturated Fat (grams)	2.1

Herb Roasted Chicken and Potatoes

SERVES 4
4 tablespoons light margarine
2 tablespoons finely chopped parsley
1/2 teaspoon ground pepper
1/2 teaspoon dried thyme
1 teaspoon dried tarragon
1 teaspoon paprika
1-1/2 pounds skinless boneless chicken breast
4 medium size baking potatoes, peeled and quartered
1 lemon

1. *Melt margarine in a measuring cup; add next 5 ingredients.*
2. *Squeeze juice of lemon over chicken.*
3. *Wash and dry potatoes; brush with margarine mixture.*
4. *Place potatoes at one end of baking dish.*
5. *Brush chicken with remaining margarine mixture and place next to potatoes.*
6. *Roast in 400 oven approximately 40 minutes, basting chicken and potatoes every 10 minutes.*

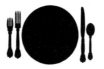

☑ Nutrition Information

Calories	376
Carbohydrates (grams)	45
Proteins (grams)	29
Cholesterol (milligrams)	69
Sodium (milligrams)	203
Fat (grams)	8.7
Saturated Fat (grams)	1.9

Sole a L'Anglaise

SERVES 4
1-1/2 pound fillets of sole
Pepper
2 tablespoons flour
1/4 cup egg substitute
1 tablespoon skim milk
1 cup dry white cracker crumbs (25 crackers)
2 teaspoons canola oil
Non-stick cooking spray

1. *Season fillets with pepper; dust with flour.*
2. *Stir milk gently into egg substitute.*
3. *Dip each fillet into mixture then coat with breadcrumbs.*
4. *Allow fillets to stand at room temperature for 15 minutes.*
5. *Spray fillets with nonstick spray.*
6. *Heat oil in non-stick skillet; saute fillets over medium heat about 4 minutes each side.*

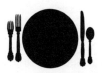

☑ Nutrition Information

Calories	264
Carbohydrates (grams)	16
Proteins (grams)	31
Cholesterol (milligrams)	80
Sodium (milligrams)	387
Fat (grams)	7.8
Saturated Fat (grams)	0.7

Spicy Sole Fillets

SERVES 4
4 tablespoons flour
4 tablespoons cornstarch
1/2 teaspoon ground coriander
1 teaspoon chili powder
1/4 teaspoon ground black pepper
1/4 teaspoon ground cloves
1/4 teaspoon ground cardamom
2 tablespoons tarragon vinegar
6 tablespoons water
1-1/3 pounds fillet of sole, cut into 12-16 pieces
1 tablespoon canola oil

1. *Combine all dry ingredients in a bowl and stir well.*
2. *Blend in vinegar and water.*
3. *Coat fillets with spice mixture.*
4. *In a nonstick skillet heat oil over medium heat.*
5. *Add fillets to oil and saute until brown on both sides.*

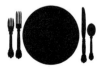

 Nutrition Information

Calories	211
Carbohydrates (grams)	13
Proteins (grams)	26
Cholesterol (milligrams)	71
Sodium (milligrams)	110
Fat (grams)	5
Saturated Fat (grams)	0.6

Chicken and Artichoke Hearts

SERVES 4
1-1/4 pound skinless boneless chicken breast
Pepper and paprika
1/4 cup dry white wine or vermouth
1 clove garlic, minced
1 large onion, chopped
2 large tomatoes, peeled, seeded and dried
1/2 teaspoon each; rosemary, thyme
1/4 teaspoon freshly ground pepper
2 cans (4-ounce) artichoke hearts, rinsed and drained
1 tablespoon cornstarch
1/2 cup, nonfat, plain yogurt

1. *Preheat oven to 425. Season chicken with pepper and paprika.*
2. *Bake uncovered in a nonstick baking pan for 5 minutes.*
3. *In a large nonstick skillet, simmer wine, garlic and onion approximately 5 minutes, over medium heat.*
4. *Add tomatoes, rosemary, thyme, pepper and chicken to skillet.*
5. *Reduce oven to 350, cover skillet and place in oven for 30 minutes. Add artichoke hearts and cook 10 minutes longer.*
6. *Drain reserving 1/2 cup liquid.*
7. *Blend cornstarch and nonfat yogurt in a saucepan.*
8. *Slowly stir in reserved liquid and simmer over low heat until heated through (be sure not to boil).*
9. *Spoon sauce over chicken and serve.*

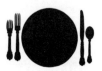

☑ Nutrition Information

Calories	208
Carbohydrates (grams)	17
Proteins (grams)	25
Cholesterol (milligrams)	58
Sodium (milligrams)	121
Fat (grams)	2.9
Saturated Fat (grams)	0.7

Mexican Chicken

SERVES 4
1-1/4 pound skinless, boneless chicken breast
1/4 cup orange juice
2 tablespoons honey
2 tablespoons dry sherry
1 clove garlic, minced
1/2 teaspoon cinnamon
1/4 teaspoon chile powder
Dash cayenne pepper

1. *Place chicken in a nonstick baking pan.*
2. *Add remaining ingredients; cover and marinate in refrigerator for 4 hours, turning occasionally.*
3. *Thirty minutes prior to baking remove from refrigerator.*
4. *Bake with marinade at 375, uncovered for approximately 50 minutes.*

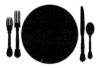

☑ *Nutrition Information*

Calories	160
Carbohydrates (grams)	11
Proteins (grams)	21
Cholesterol (milligrams)	57
Sodium (milligrams)	50
Fat (grams)	2.4
Saturated Fat (grams)	0.6

Chili Con Carne

SERVES 4-6
1 pound lean ground turkey
3/4 cup chopped onion
3/4 cup chopped green pepper
1 can (16-ounce) whole tomatoes, crushed
1 can (15-ounce) kidney beans, undrained
1 can (8-ounce) tomato puree
1 tablespoon chile powder
1/2 tablespoon cumin
Pepper to taste

1. *In a nonstick skillet, brown turkey, onion and pepper over medium-high heat.*
2. *Drain off fat.*
3. *Add remaining ingredients and bring to a boil.*
4. *Reduce heat; cover and simmer approximately 2 hours.*

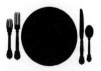

☑ _Nutrition Information_

Calories	203
Carbohydrates (grams)	22
Proteins (grams)	16
Cholesterol (milligrams)	28
Sodium (milligrams)	397
Fat (grams)	6.2
Saturated Fat (grams)	1.9

Bombay Shrimp

SERVES 6
1-1/2 pounds large shrimp, peeled and deveined
1 tablespoon all-purpose flour
2 teaspoons vegetable oil
1/2 cup minced shallots
1 tablespoon curry powder
1 cup diced red bell pepper
1-1/2 cups diced tomato
1/2 cup light coconut milk
1/4 cup chopped fresh or 4 teaspoons dried basil
1 tablespoon lemon fresh juice
1 teaspoon sugar
1/2 teaspoon salt
1 (10-1/2 ounce) can low-salt chicken broth
6 cups hot cooked rice
3 tablespoons flaked sweetened coconut, toasted

1. *In a bowl toss together shrimp and flour; set aside.*
2. *In a nonstick skillet over medium-high heat, saute shallots curry powder and bell pepper approximately 2 minutes.*
3. *Add tomato and next 6 ingredients; simmer and cook 2 minutes.*
4. *Add shrimp and simmer 4 minutes stirring occasionally.*
5. *Spoon shrimp and sauce over rice; top with coconut.*

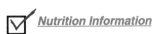
Nutrition Information

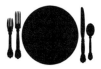

Calories	397
Carbohydrates (grams)	61.2
Proteins (grams)	23.2
Cholesterol (milligrams)	129
Sodium (milligrams)	361
Fat (grams)	6
Saturated Fat (grams)	2.1

Stuffed Poblano Chiles

SERVES 2
2 large poblano chiles (about 8 ounces)
2 large tomatilloes • Vegetable cooking spray
1/3 cup chopped red bell pepper
1/4 cup chopped green onions • 1 garlic clove, crushed
2 tablespoons chopped fresh cilantro
1/2 teaspoon chili powder
1/4 teaspoon ground cumin • 1/4 teaspoon pepper
1 cup drained canned black beans, divided
1 cup shredded cooked chicken breast
1/3 cup frozen whole-kernel corn, thawed
1/4 cup nonfat sour cream
1/4 cup (1 ounce) shredded reduced-fat Monterey Jack
cheese, divided

1. Preheat oven to 400.
2. Cut chiles in two lengthwise; remove seeds and membranes; set aside. Remove husks from tomatilloes; chop well.
3. Coat a nonstick skillet with nonstick spray and place over medium-high heat.
4. Add tomatilloes, bell pepper onion and garlic; saute 3 minutes.
5. Remove from heat and stir in cilantro, chili powder, cumin and pepper; set aside.
6. Mash 1/2 cup beans in a bowl.
7. Stir in remaining beans, bell pepper mixture, chicken, corn, nonfat sour cream and 2 tablespoons cheese.
8. Stuff each chile half with bean mixture; top with remaining 2 tablespoons cheese and bake at 400 for 20 minutes.

☑ **Nutrition Information**

Calories	387
Carbohydrates (grams)	46.8
Proteins (grams)	38.3
Cholesterol (milligrams)	64
Sodium (milligrams)	363
Fat (grams)	6.9
Saturated Fat (grams)	2.3

Mexican Veal Stew

SERVES 4
1 (2-pound) boneless veal leg roast
3-1/2 cups low-salt chicken broth
1 cup sliced carrot
3/4 cup sliced celery
1/2 cup thinly sliced green onions
1/3 cup thinly sliced seeded jalapeno pepper
1/3 cup fresh cilantro leaves
6 garlic cloves
1 bay leaf
1/2 cup orange juice
1/4 cup fresh lemon juice
1/2 teaspoon salt

1. *Combine fat-trimmed roast and broth and next 7 ingredients in a Dutch oven. Boil, then remove from heat.*
2. *Bake, covered at 325 until roast is tender (about 1 - 1-1/2 hours). Remove roast from pan and reserve liquid and vegetables.*
3. *Let roast cool for 10 minutes. Shred roast with fork; set aside.*
4. *Discard bay leaf from reserved liquid. Puree liquid and vegetables in a blender until smooth; return puree to pan.*
5. *Add fruit juices and boil; cook until mixture is reduced to 2 cups.*
6. *Place shredded roast in pan; add salt.*
7. *Cook over medium heat until thoroughly heated.*

☑ Nutrition Information

Calories	323
Carbohydrates (grams)	14.8
Proteins (grams)	52.1
Cholesterol (milligrams)	177
Sodium (milligrams)	544
Fat (grams)	5.6
Saturated Fat (grams)	1.3

Spiced Turkey with Peaches

SERVES 4
1 3/4 pounds turkey breast cutlets
1 teaspoon ground cinnamon
4 tablespoons flour
1 teaspoon ground cloves
1 tablespoon light margarine
2/3 cup finely chopped onion
4 teaspoon sugar
2 tablespoon fresh lemon juice
1/2 cup water
1 cup frozen peach slices
1 teaspoon diet margarine
1/2 cup nonfat sour cream

1. *Combine cinnamon, cloves and flour.*
2. *Dredge turkey in flour mixture, coating both sides well.*
3. *Heat 1 tablespoon diet margarine in a nonstick skillet; add turkey and brown over medium heat.*
4. *Add onions to skillet and cook approximately 2 minutes.*
5. *Sprinkle turkey with sugar and lemon juice; top turkey with onions. Add water; cover and simmer over low heat for 30 minutes, basting turkey halfway through.*
6. *Melt 1 teaspoon diet margarine in a skillet; add peach slices and coat well with margarine.*
7. *About 3 minutes prior to when turkey is done, heat peaches until hot.*
8. *Spoon peaches over turkey and top with a dollop of nonfat sour cream.*

Nutrition Information

Calories	361
Carbohydrates (grams)	35
Proteins (grams)	42
Cholesterol (milligrams)	87
Sodium (milligrams)	174
Fat (grams)	4.6
Saturated Fat (grams)	2.3

Ham, Apricots and Bananas

SERVES 4
2 tablespoons light margarine
1/2 teaspoon ground cinnamon
1 teaspoon curry powder
2 tablespoons (packed) light brown sugar
2 tablespoons fresh lemon juice
4 tablespoons mango chutney, solid
pieces, finely chopped
2 fully cooked ham slices (3/4 pound each) 1/4 inch thick
2 cans (8-ounce each) apricot halves, drained
2 small, ripe bananas

1. Melt margarine and remove from heat.
2. Add chutney curry powder, brown sugar and lemon juice.
3. Trim fat from ham and cut ham in half; place in baking dish.
4. Peel bananas and slice.
5. Place apricot halves and banana slices atop ham.
6. Pour chutney mixture over apricots and bananas.
7. Broil until lightly browned.

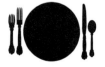

☑ *Nutrition Information*

Calories	412
Proteins (grams)	29
Cholesterol (milligrams)	71
Sodium (milligrams)	1903
Fat (grams)	14
Saturated Fat (grams)	4.3

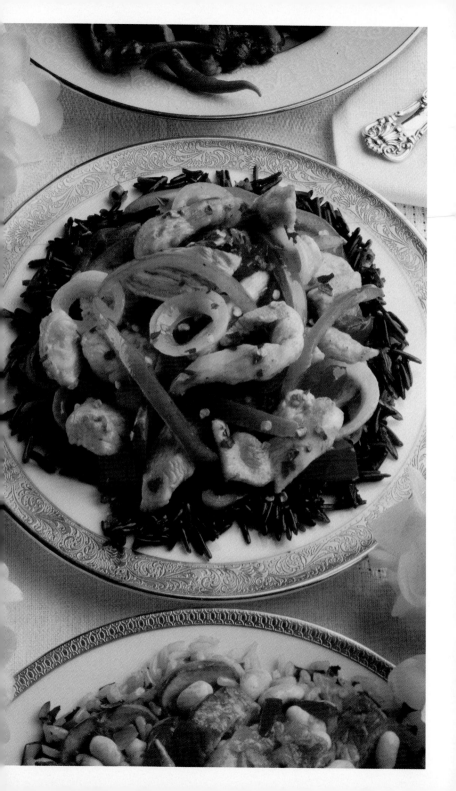

Chicken Cacciatore

Everyone loves this classic cacciatore. Serve over rice for a complete meal.

Photo Credits
Photography by Barney Taxel
Barney Taxel & Co.
216/431-2400

Recipe Credits
Chicken Cacciatore, see page 61
Servings: 4

Middle Eastern Fattoush

SERVES 6
2 whole-wheat pita breads, store bought
Juice of 2 lemons
2 garlic cloves, minced or put through a press
Freshly ground pepper
1/2 cup plain nonfat yogurt
1 large or 2 small cucumbers, chopped or 1 small head
romaine lettuce, leaves washed and cut into 1 inch pieces
1 medium sized red onion, chopped
1 pound (4 to 5) firm, ripe tomatoes, chopped
1 green pepper, chopped (optional)
1 bunch parsley, finely chopped
2 tablespoons chopped fresh mint
3 tablespoons chopped cilantro

1. *Cut pitas in half and toast until crisp.*
2. *Break into small pieces and place in a salad bowl.*
3. *Combine lemon juice, garlic, pepper and nonfat yogurt; toss with pita pieces.*
4. *Add vegetables and herbs; toss again.*
5. *Adjust seasonings and serve.*

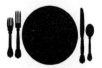

☑ *Nutrition Information*

Calories	75
Carbohydrates (grams)	15
Proteins (grams)	3.8
Cholesterol (milligrams)	0.4
Sodium (milligrams)	91
Fat (grams)	0.5
Saturated Fat (grams)	0

Spanish Tortilla

SERVES 4
1 large russet potato (5-6 ounces), scrubbed and diced
1 teaspoon olive oil
1/2 medium-sized onion (2 ounces) chopped
Freshly ground pepper
1-1/2 cup egg substitute

1. *Steam potato approximately 8 minutes or until crisp yet tender.*
2. *In a nonstick skillet, heat oil and saute onion until tender.*
3. *Stir in potatoes.*
4. *Pour in egg substitute and add pepper to taste; make sure egg substitute is distributed evenly around skillet.*
5. *Over low heat, cook, covered, about 10 minutes or until eggs are set.*
6. *Preheat broiler.*
7. *Uncover pan and place under broiler about 2-3 minutes.*
8. *Allow to cool to room temperature; cut into wedges and serve.*

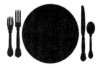

Nutrition Information

Calories	124
Carbohydrates (grams)	8
Proteins (grams)	12
Cholesterol (milligrams)	0.9
Sodium (milligrams)	170
Fat (grams)	4.3
Saturated Fat (grams)	0.8

Black-Eyed Pea
and Tomato Salad

SERVES 4
1 cup dried black-eyed peas, washed
1/2 small onion, chopped
2 large garlic cloves, minced or pressed
1 quart water • 1 bay leaf
2 large ripe tomatoes, diced
1 to 2 green chili peppers, seeded and minced
2 cups fresh spinach, chopped
Dressing: 5 tablespoons fresh lemon juice
1/2 teaspoon ground cumin
1 small garlic clove, minced
1/2 cup plain nonfat yogurt
Ground pepper to taste

1. *Combine peas, onion, garlic, water and bayleaf; boil.*
2. *Cover and simmer over low heat for 30 minutes until beans are thoroughly cooked but not mushy.*
3. *Drain; discard bay leaf.*
4. *Toss together beans, tomatoes and chili peppers.*
5. *For dressing: Combine lemon juice, cumin, garlic nonfat yogurt and pepper to taste. Mix salad with dressing and chill several hours.*
6. *Just before serving add spinach; toss and serve.*

☑ **Nutrition Information**

Calories	145
Carbohydrates (grams)	30
Proteins (grams)	5.1
Cholesterol (milligrams)	0
Sodium (milligrams)	17
Fat (grams)	0.8
Saturated Fat (grams)	0.2

Turkish Shrimp with Cumin

SERVES 6
1-1/2 pounds shrimp in their shells
3 cups water
2 strips lemon zest
4 parsley sprigs
2 garlic cloves, crushed
6 peppercorns
1 tablespoon olive oil
1 large onion, chopped
4 additional garlic cloves, minced
1 to 1-1/2 teaspoon ground cumin
Pinch of cayenne pepper
Freshly ground pepper
2 to 3 tablespoons chopped cilantro
cooked rice for serving

1. *Peel shrimp. In a saucepan combine shells, water, lemon zest, parsley, 2 garlic cloves, peppercorns and celery leaves; bring to a boil, then simmer over medium heat 45 minutes.*
2. *Strain mixture and reserve 1 cup liquid.*
3. *In a large nonstick skillet, heat oil and saute onion and 4 garlic cloves; add cumin, cayenne pepper and ground pepper to taste.*
4. *Add shrimp. Stir in reserved liquid and bring to a boil.*
5. *Reduce heat and simmer 10 minutes.*
6. *Sprinkle with cilantro; serve over rice.*

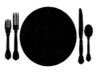

☑ *Nutrition Information*

Calories	128
Carbohydrates (grams)	0
Proteins (grams)	19
Cholesterol (milligrams)	174
Sodium (milligrams)	199
Fat (grams)	5.5
Saturated Fat (grams)	1.2

Grilled Swordfish with Lemon and Garlic

SERVES 4
4 (1/2 inch-thick) swordfish steaks, 6 ounces each
2 teaspoons olive oil
Freshly ground pepper
1 to 2 garlic cloves, minced
6 tablespoons fresh lemon juice

---

1. *Preheat grill.*
2. *Brush swordfish with 1 teaspoon olive oil and pepper.*
3. *Combine minced garlic, lemon juice and remaining olive oil; blend together well.*
4. *Grill fish; remove from heat.*
5. *Spoon lemon mixture over each steak and serve.*

☑ Nutrition Information

Calories	226
Carbohydrates (grams)	0
Proteins (grams)	34
Cholesterol (milligrams)	67
Sodium (milligrams)	153
Fat (grams)	9
Saturated Fat (grams)	2.2

Moroccan Grilled Snapper

SERVES 4
12 garlic cloves
1 bunch cilantro
1 tablespoon paprika
1 tablespoon ground cumin
Pinch of cayenne pepper
Juice of 2 large lemons
1 teaspoon olive oil
4 to 6 ounce snapper steaks

1. Mash together garlic, cilantro, paprika, cumin and cayenne pepper; stir in lemon juice and olive oil.
2. Marinate snapper in mixture for several hours.
3. Grill fish, basting halfway through.
4. Serve immediately.

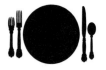

☑ Nutrition Information

Calories	228
Carbohydrates (grams)	0
Proteins (grams)	45
Cholesterol (milligrams)	80
Sodium (milligrams)	96
Fat (grams)	4
Saturated Fat (grams)	0.8

Italian Bean and Tuna Salad

SERVES 4
1 red onion, very thinly sliced
3 to 4 tablespoons red wine vinegar
2 cups cooked white beans
1 6-1/2 ounce can water-packed tuna, drained
2 tomatoes, diced
1 garlic clove, minced
Juice of 1 lemon
3 to 4 tablespoons chopped, fresh basil or parsley
1 teaspoon chopped fresh sage
1 tablespoon olive oil
1 tablespoon plain nonfat yogurt
Freshly ground pepper
Romaine lettuce leaves

1. Toss onion with 2 tablespoons vinegar; add water and soak 30 minutes; drain.
2. Toss onion with remaining ingredients except lettuce.
3. Line serving plates with lettuce; top with salad.

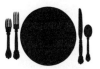

☑ *Nutrition Information*

Calories	222
Carbohydrates (grams)	23
Proteins (grams)	21
Cholesterol (milligrams)	19
Sodium (milligrams)	185
Fat (grams)	5
Saturated Fat (grams)	0.9

Stir Fry Scallops and Vegetables

SERVES 4
4 teaspoons canola oil (divided)
1 pound scallops • 1 teaspoon minced garlic
1 teaspoon minced fresh ginger
2 small (3 ounce) carrots, peeled and sliced diagonally,
1/8 inch thick
2 stalk celery, sliced diagonally 1/4 inch thick
1/4 pounds (30 small) snow peas, tips and
strings removed
2/3 cup thin green onion • 4 tablespoons water
Seasoning mixture:
3 teaspoons cornstarch
1/2 teaspoon sugar
2 tablespoons low sodium soy sauce
3 tablespoons oyster sauce • 6 tablespoons water
1 teaspoon oriental sesame oil

1. *Blend together all ingredients for seasoning mixture; set aside.*
2. *Heat a wok; add 2 teaspoons oil to heated wok and immediately add scallops, garlic and ginger.*
3. *Stir fry 3 minutes; remove scallops.*
4. *Add 2 teaspoons oil to wok and immediately add carrot and celery slices; stir-fry 30 seconds.*
5. *Add snow peas and green onion to wok; stir-fry 30 seconds.*
6. *Add 4 tablespoons water to wok, cover and steam about 2 minutes.*
7. *Return scallops to wok; add seasoning mixture; stir and cook until liquid thickens.*

☑ *Nutrition Information*

Calories	200
Carbohydrates (grams)	14
Proteins (grams)	20
Cholesterol (milligrams)	40
Sodium (milligrams)	780
Fat (grams)	6.7
Saturated Fat (grams)	0.7

Lamb Chops, Peppers and Tomato in Spicy Sauce

SERVES 4
8 loin lamb chops - 1 inch thick
3 tablespoons soy sauce
2 small onions, peeled, quartered, layers separated
1 medium size green pepper, cut in 1 inch squares
1/2 cup water, divided
2 small tomatoes
2 tablespoons light brown sugar
2 tablespoons curry powder
1/2 cup catsup
2 tablespoons oyster sauce
Non stick cooking spray

1. Trim fat from lamb chops; season with soy sauce.
2. Coat a nonstick pan with nonstick cooking spray; saute onions and peppers about 2 minutes.
3. Add 4 tablespoons water, cover and steam about 3 minutes.
4. Uncover pan and let liquid evaporate.
5. Remove onion and pepper.
6. Add lamb chops to pan and brown over medium heat, about 4 minutes each side.
7. Cut each tomato in quarters; toss with brown sugar; set aside.
8. Remove lamb chops from pan.
9. Add curry powder and liquid to pan; turn heat to low and add 4 tablespoons water, catsup and oyster sauce.
10. Add onion, pepper and tomato quarters; heat through and spoon over lamb.

Nutrition Information

Calories	285
Carbohydrates (grams)	17
Proteins (grams)	33
Cholesterol (milligrams)	102
Sodium (milligrams)	1165
Fat (grams)	9
Saturated Fat (grams)	3.3

Chicken, Garlic and Vegetables

SERVES 4
8 small skinless chicken thighs
1/2 teaspoon ground black pepper, divided
1 tablespoon light margarine
4 small red-skinned potatoes
4 medium size carrots
16 large cloves garlic
1 teaspoon dried basil
1/2 cup chicken broth
1/2 cup frozen green peas
1/2 cup frozen corn
4 slices crusty french bread

---

1. Season chicken with pepper.
2. Melt diet margarine in nonstick skillet and brown chicken over medium-high heat.
3. Quarter potatoes; peel carrots and slice diagonally.
4. Separate garlic cloves but do not peel.
5. Remove chicken from skillet.
6. Add potatoes, garlic and carrots to skillet; sprinkle with 1/4 teaspoon pepper and basil; stir.
7. Return chicken to skillet atop vegetables.
8. Pour in chicken broth; cover and simmer about 25 minutes.
9. Add peas and corn to skillet; simmer 5 minutes.
10. Remove garlic and serve separately; to eat garlic squeeze cloves to remove skin and spread on bread.

☑ **Nutrition Information**

Calories	460
Carbohydrates (grams)	51
Proteins (grams)	33
Cholesterol (milligrams)	95
Sodium (milligrams)	499
Fat (grams)	14
Saturated Fat (grams)	3.7

Cointreau Chicken

SERVES 4
3 cups water
4 small carrots, peeled and sliced diagonally
1-1/3 pounds skinless, boneless chicken breast
3 tablespoons flour
1/4 teaspoon ground pepper
4 tablespoons light margarine
1/2 cup cointreau
1 teaspoon grated orange peel
1/2 cup canned condensed chicken broth
2 cups seedless green grapes

1. Boil water; add carrots and cover; simmer until carrots are tender; drain.
2. Cut chicken breasts in half. Combine flour and pepper in a bag.
3. Melt 2 tablespoons diet margarine in a nonstick pan.
4. Add chicken to bag with flour mixture and shake to coat pieces.
5. Brown in diet margarine. Pour Cointreau over chicken; turn to glaze. Remove chicken to serving dish.
6. Add chicken broth and orange peel to pan; boil down to 6 tablespoons; add remaining 2 tablespoons diet margarine.
7. Add carrot; heat 1 minute.
8. Add grapes and heat 2 minutes more.
9. Arrange carrots and grapes around chicken and top with remaining sauce.

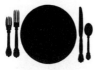

☑ Nutrition Information

Calories	260
Carbohydrates (grams)	20
Proteins (grams)	25
Cholesterol (milligrams)	61
Sodium (milligrams)	404
Fat (grams)	9
Saturated Fat (grams)	1.9

Moroccan Beef

SERVES 6

1-1/2 pounds lean round steak
1/2 teaspoon ground coriander
1/2 teaspoon ground cumin
1/4 teaspoon ground ginger
1/4 teaspoon pepper
1/8 teaspoon saffron threads, crushed
Olive oil-flavored vegetable cooking spray
2 cups sliced carrot
1 medium onion, sliced
1/2 cup water
1/4 cup lemon juice
2 tablespoons chopped fresh parsley
1 tablespoon chopped fresh mint
1/2 teaspoon chicken-flavored bouillon granules
2 cups cooked couscous (cooked without salt or fat)
Grated lemon rind (optional)
Chopped fresh parsley (optional)

1. *Trim fat from steak; cut into bite-size pieces and place in baking dish. Combine next 5 ingredients in a bowl and stir well.*
2. *Season steak with spice mixture; cover and refrigerate 8 hours.*
3. *Coat a Dutch oven with nonstick cooking spray; heat until hot.*
4. *Add steak and brown, stirring often.*
5. *Add carrot and next 6 ingredients; boil; cover and simmer over low heat about 1 hour.*
6. *Place cooked couscous on serving platter; spoon beef over couscous. Garnish with optional ingredients.*

☑ **Nutrition Information**

Calories	255
Carbohydrates (grams)	21.0
Proteins (grams)	28.2
Cholesterol (milligrams)	66
Sodium (milligrams)	148
Fat (grams)	6.0
Saturated Fat (grams)	1.8

Swordfish Calcutta

SERVES 4
2 tablespoons unsweetened orange juice
1 tablespoon lemon juice
1/2 teaspoon ground coriander
1/2 teaspoon ground cumin
1/4 teaspoon ground cardamom
1/4 teaspoon ground cinnamon
1/4 teaspoon ground nutmeg
1/8 teaspoon ground cloves
1/8 teaspoon pepper
4 (4-ounce) swordfish steaks (3/4-inch thick)
Vegetable cooking spray

1. Combine first 9 ingredients in a bowl; stir well.
2. Place swordfish in a baking pan; brush with orange juice mixture; cover and marinate 8 hours.
3. Broil swordfish, discarding marinade, about 10-12 minutes.

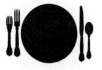

 Nutrition Information

Calories	155
Carbohydrates (grams)	0.9
Proteins (grams)	24.4
Cholesterol (milligrams)	48
Sodium (milligrams)	111
Fat (grams)	5.3
Saturated Fat (grams)	1.2

Thai-Style Flounder

SERVES 4
3 cups boiling water
2 tablespoons minced peeled gingerroot
1/2 teaspoon coriander seeds
3 regular-size oolang tea bags
1 (3-inch) strip lemon rind
4 (6-ounce) skinned flounder fillets
1 cup (2-inch) sliced green onions
1 cup (1/4-inch) diagonally sliced carrot
1/4 cup minced shallots
Thai Scallion Sauce:
1/2 cup low-sodium soy sauce • 1/4 cup fish sauce
2 tablespoons thinly sliced green onions
1 tablespoon chopped fresh cilantro
2 tablespoons rice vinegar • 2 teaspoons sugar
1 teaspoon chopped fresh mint
1 teaspoon dark sesame oil
1/2 teaspoon minced peeled gingerroot
1/4 teaspoon chili-and-garlic paste
1 garlic clove, minced

1. *Combine water, gingerroot, coriander, tea bags and lemon rind in a bowl; let stand 1 hour.*
2. *Roll each fillet jelly-roll fashion and place in an nonstick skillet.*
3. *Add green onion, carrot and shallots.*
4. *Strain tea mixture into skillet and boil.*
5. *Reduce heat and simmer, uncovered, about 8 minutes.*
6. *Remove fish and vegetables to serving platter; serve with thai-scallion sauce.*
7. *Sauce: Combine all ingredients in a bowl and stir well.*

☑ **Nutrition Information**

Calories	191
Carbohydrates (grams)	7.4
Proteins (grams)	33.1
Cholesterol (milligrams)	0
Sodium (milligrams)	475
Fat (grams)	0.2
Saturated Fat (grams)	0

Chicken Cha Cha

SERVES 4

2 tablespoons olive oil
2 teaspoons minced garlic (2 medium cloves)
4 boneless, skinless chicken breast halves (about 1 lb.)
1/2 teaspoon salt, or to taste
1/8 teaspoon ground cumin
Freshly-ground black pepper, to taste
1 large green bell pepper, stemmed, seeded and cut
lengthwise into thin julienne strips
1 large red bell pepper, stemmed, seeded and cut lengthwise into thin julienne strips
1 large yellow bell pepper, stemmed, seeded and cut
lengthwise into thin julienne strips
1 teaspoon granulated sugar
2 large oranges, peeled, cut lengthwise into thin slices

1. *In a nonstick skillet, heat oil over medium heat.*
2. *Add garlic and cook 1 minute.*
3. *Add chicken breasts and brown well on both sides.*
4. *Season with salt, cumin and pepper to taste.*
5. *Add pepper strips and sugar.*
6. *Cover and simmer about 5 minutes.*
7. *Add orange slices and heat through.*

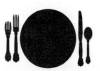

☑ Nutrition Information

Calories	260
Carbohydrates (grams)	28
Proteins (grams)	19
Cholesterol (milligrams)	45
Sodium (milligrams)	43
Fat (grams)	9
Saturated Fat (grams)	1.6

Beef Bourguignonne

SERVES 6
1 lb. boneless beef chuck roast, cut into 3/4-inch cubes
2 teaspoons cooking oil • 1 cup chopped onion
1 clove garlic, minced • 1-1/2 cups burgundy
3/4 cup beef broth • 2 bay leaves
1 teaspoon dried thyme, crushed
3/4 teaspoon dried marjoram, crushed
1/4 teaspoon pepper
3 cups fresh mushrooms
4 medium carrots, cut into 3/4-inch pieces
1/2 lb. pearl onions or 2 cups small frozen whole onions
1/4 cup cold water
2 tablespoons all-purpose flour
3 cups hot cooked noodles

1. *Heat 1 teaspoon oil in a large Dutch oven; add half the meat and brown. Remove the meat from pan; add remaining oil and meat, chopped onion and garlic.*
2. *Brown remaining meat; drain fat; return all meat to Dutch oven.*
3. *Stir in burgundy, beef broth, bay leaves, marjoram and pepper; boil then reduce heat and simmer, covered, 40 minutes.*
4. *Add mushrooms, carrots and pearl onions; return to boil then reduce heat, cover and cook 30 minutes more.*
5. *Combine water and flour; stir into meat mixture until thickened and bubbly.*
6. *Serve over noodles.*

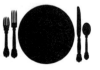

☑ Nutrition Information

Calories	434
Carbohydrates (grams)	36
Proteins (grams)	30
Cholesterol (milligrams)	80
Sodium (milligrams)	396
Fat (grams)	14
Saturated Fat (grams)	5

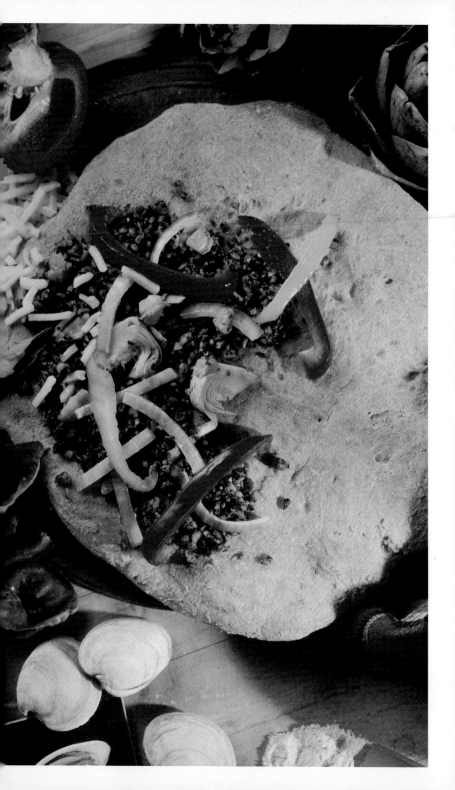

Pesto-Onion-Pepper Pizza

Quick, easy and light fare for the entire family.

Photo Credits
Photography by Barney Taxel
Barney Taxel & Co.
216/431-2400

Recipe Credits
Pesto-Onion-Pepper Pizza, see page 62
Servings: 8 slices

Citrus Lobster Salad

SERVES 4

3 (8-ounce) fresh or frozen lobster tails, thawed
1 medium-size pink grapefruit, peeled and sectioned
1 medium-size orange, peeled and sectioned
1/4 cup orange low-fat yogurt
3 tablespoons orange juice
1 tablespoon fresh lemon juice
1 teaspoon grated orange rind
1 teaspoon grated lime rind
1/8 teaspoon ground white pepper
4 cups torn fresh spinach
2 teaspoons chopped fresh chives

1. Boil water and cook lobster tails 6-8 minutes or until done.
2. Rinse with cold water. Split and clean tails.
3. Cut lobster meat int bite-size pieces.
4. Combine lobster, grapefruit and orange sections.
5. In a small bowl combine yogurt, orange juice, lemon juice, orange rind, lime rind, and pepper; stir well.
6. Pour mixture over lobster and toss well.
7. Arrange spinach on serving plates; top with lobster salad; sprinkle with chives.

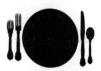

☑ Nutrition Information

Calories	153
Carbohydrates (grams)	11.6
Proteins (grams)	24.3
Cholesterol (milligrams)	80
Sodium (milligrams)	444
Fat (grams)	1.0
Saturated Fat (grams)	0.2

French-Style Veal Shanks

SERVES 4
4 (5-ounce) veal shanks
Vegetable cooking spray
1 (14-1/2-ounce) can of no-salt-added whole tomatoes,
undrained and chopped
1/4 cup Chablis or other dry white wine
1/4 cup sliced ripe olives
1 tablespoon grated orange rind
2 teaspoons dried whole tarragon
1/4 teaspoon salt
1/4 teaspoon pepper
Minced fresh parsley (optional)

1. Trim fat from shanks.
2. Coat a large nonstick skillet with cooking spray.
3. Place over medium-high heat until hot.
4. Add shanks and cook 3 minutes on each side or until browned.
5. Combine tomato and next 6 ingredients in a medium bowl; pour over shanks.
6. Cover and bake at 325 degrees for 1-1/2 hours or until shanks are tender.
7. Transfer to a serving platter with a slotted spoon.
8. Garnish with minced fresh parsley, if desired.

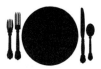

☑ Nutrition Information

Calories	175
Carbohydrates (grams)	5.9
Proteins (grams)	22.1
Cholesterol (milligrams)	94
Sodium (milligrams)	302
Fat (grams)	7.0
Saturated Fat (grams)	2.6

Greek Stuffed Steak

SERVES 8
1/3 cup finely chopped red onion
1/3 cup chopped pickled pepperoncini peppers
2 tablespoons dry breadcrumbs
1/4 teaspoon salt
1/4 teaspoon garlic powder
1 (10-ounce) package frozen chopped spinach, thawed,
drained, and squeezed dry
1 (1-1/2-pound) lean flank steak
Vegetable cooking spray
1/2 cup water • 1/2 cup dry red wine
1/2 teaspoon dried oregano

1. *Combine first 6 ingredients in a bowl; stir well, and set aside.*
2. *Trim fat from steak. Using a sharp knife, cut horizontally through center of steak, cutting to, but not through, other side; open flat as you would a book.*
3. *Place steak between 2 sheets of heavy-duty plastic wrap, and flatten to an even thickness, using a meat mallet or rolling   pin.*
4. *Spread spinach mixture over steak, leaving a 1-inch margin around outside edges.*
5. *Roll up steak, jelly-roll fashion, starting with short side. Secure at 2-inch intervals with heavy string.*
6. *Coat oven with cooking spray, and place over medium-high heat until hot. Add steak, browning well on all sides.*
7. *Add water, wine, and oregano to pan; bring to a boil.*
8. *Cover, reduce heat, and simmer 1 hour or until tender.*
9. *Remove string, and cut steak into 16 slices. Serve with cooking liquid.*

☑ Nutrition Information

Calories	160
Carbohydrates (grams)	4.4
Proteins (grams)	17.6
Cholesterol (milligrams)	40
Sodium (milligrams)	261
Fat (grams)	7.9
Saturated Fat (grams)	3.3

California Seafood Stew

SERVES 6
Vegetable cooking spray
1/2 cup chopped onion
1/2 cup chopped sweet red pepper
1 clove garlic, minced
1 (14 1/2-ounce) can no-salt-added whole tomatoes,
undrained and chopped
1 (8-ounce) can no-salt-added tomato sauce
1/4 cup Burgundy or other dry red wine
1/4 cup chopped fresh oregano
2 tablespoons chopped fresh parsley
1 teaspoon low-sodium Worcestershire sauce
1/4 teaspoon crushed red pepper
1/2 pound bay scallops
1/2 lb. medium-size fresh shrimp, peeled and deveined
1 (10-ounce) can whole baby clams, drained

1. *Place a Dutch oven over medium-high heat; coat with nonstick spray.*
2. *Add onion red pepper and garlic and saute until tender.*
3. *Add tomato, tomato sauce and Burgundy; stir well.*
4. *Add next 4 ingredients and stir well.*
5. *Bring mixture to a boil;cover; simmer over low heat 20 minutes.*
6. *Add seafood; bring to a boil.*
7. *Reduce heat; simmer until scallops and shrimp are done (8-10 minutes).*

☑ Nutrition Information

Calories	146
Carbohydrates (grams)	11.5
Proteins (grams)	20.9
Cholesterol (milligrams)	77
Sodium (milligrams)	160
Fat (grams)	1.6
Saturated Fat (grams)	0.3

Gumbo

SERVES 8
1 pound fresh or frozen fish fillets
1 pound fresh or frozen shrimp in shells
1/2 cup all-purpose flour
1/4 cup cooking oil and 1/4 cup water
1 large onion, chopped (1 cup)
2 stalks celery, chopped (1 cup)
1 medium green pepper, chopped (3/4 cup)
6 cloves garlic, minced • 6 cups chicken broth
2 cups sliced okra or one 10-oz. package frozen cut okra
3 bay leaves • 1 teaspoon dried oregano, crushed
1 teaspoon dried thyme, crushed
1 teaspoon dried basil, crushed
1/2 teaspoon ground red pepper
1/4 teaspoon ground black pepper
1 lb. smoked turkey sausage cut into 1/2-inch-thick slices
4 cups hot cooked rice

1. Make sure fish is thawed and skin removed; cut into 1-inch pieces.
2. Peel and clean shrimp; rinse and refrigerate along with fillets until ready to use.
3. In a Dutch oven, stir together flour, water and oil until smooth.
4. Stir constantly, over medium-low heat about 30 minutes.
5. Add celery, green pepper and garlic. Cook over medium heat for 10-15 minutes. Slowly stir in chicken broth.
6. Add okra and next 6 ingredients; stir well. Bring to a boil; cover; reduce heat and simmer 1 hour.
7. Add turkey sausage and simmer 10 more minutes.
8. Add fish and shrimp and simmer 5 minutes.
9. Skim off fat and serve.

☑ **Nutrition Information**

Calories	453
Carbohydrates (grams)	44
Proteins (grams)	37
Cholesterol (milligrams)	148
Sodium (milligrams)	1196
Fat (grams)	13
Saturated Fat (grams)	2.3

Scallop Combo Tropical

SERVES 6
2 medium oranges
Vegetable cooking spray
2 teaspoons vegetable oil
1-1/2 pounds fresh bay scallops
1 small green pepper, cut into strips
1 small sweet red pepper, cut into strips
1/2 cup chopped onion
1 clove garlic, minced
1 cup unsweetened orange juice
1 tablespoon cornstarch
1/2 teaspoon ground ginger
1/4 teaspoon dry mustard
1/4 teaspoon ground red pepper
1-1/2 cups cubed fresh pineapple

1. *Peel oranges and cut into 1/4 inch thick slices; set aside.*
2. *Spray a nonstick pan with cooking spray; heat oil until hot.*
3. *Add scallops and saute 2-3 minutes.*
4. *Add pepper strips, onion and garlic; saute 3 minutes.*
5. *Remove scallops and vegetables from pan; discard liquid and wipe pan clean.*
6. *Add orange juice and next 4 ingredients to pan; stir constantly over medium heat until thickened.*
7. *Add scallops and vegetables, oranges and pineapple; cook until thoroughly heated, stirring well.*

☑ **Nutrition Information**

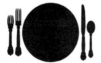

Calories	200
Carbohydrates (grams)	23
Proteins (grams)	21
Cholesterol (milligrams)	37
Sodium (milligrams)	184
Fat (grams)	2.9
Saturated Fat (grams)	1.1

German-Style Meatballs

SERVES 4
1/4 cup egg substitute
1/4 cup beer
1/4 cup fine dry bread crumbs
Dash of pepper
1 pound extra lean ground beef
2 medium onions, sliced and separated into rings
1 tablespoon canola oil
3 tablespoons all-purpose flour
1 teaspoon instant beef bouillon granules
1 teaspoon brown sugar
1/4 teaspoon dried thyme, crushed
1 cup beer
1/4 cup water
1 teaspoon vinegar
2 tablespoons snipped parsley
3 cups cooked spaghetti

1. Combine egg substitute with 1/4 cup of beer, breadcrumbs and pepper in a large bowl.
2. Add ground beef and mix well. Shape into 24 meatballs.
3. Bake meatballs in a 350 oven for 15-20 minutes.
4. In a large nonstick pan saute onions in oil until tender.
5. Stir in flour, bouillon, brown sugar and thyme.
6. Add remaining beer, water and vinegar; cook and stir until thickened.
7. Stir in parsley and meatballs; heat through.
8. Serve over spaghetti.

☑ Nutrition Information

Calories	516
Carbohydrates (grams)	48
Proteins (grams)	32
Cholesterol (milligrams)	71
Sodium (milligrams)	407
Fat (grams)	18
Saturated Fat (grams)	5.9

Irish Stew

SERVES 6

3/4 pound lean boneless lamb, cut into 1-inch cubes
2 cups beef broth
1/4 teaspoon pepper
1 bay leaf
4 medium carrots, sliced 1/2 inch thick
3 medium potatoes (1 pound), peeled and quartered
2 medium onions, cut into wedges
1/2 teaspoon dried thyme, crushed
1/2 teaspoon dried basil, crushed
1/2 cup cold water
2 tablespoons all-purpose flour
Snipped parsley

1. *Combine lamb, broth, pepper and bayleaf in a large pan; bring to a boil.*
2. *Reduce heat and simmer, covered, for 30 minutes.*
3. *Skim fat from meat mixture; add next 5 ingredients and simmer, covered, another 30 minutes.*
4. *Combine water and flour in a small bowl; add to meat mixture.*
5. *Cook, stirring constantly until mixture is thickened.*
6. *Sprinkle with parsley and serve.*

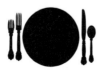

☑ *Nutrition Information*

Calories	184
Carbohydrates (grams)	24
Proteins (grams)	14
Cholesterol (milligrams)	35
Sodium (milligrams)	416
Fat (grams)	4
Saturated Fat (grams)	1

Cioppino

SERVES 4

1 pound fresh or frozen fish fillets
3/4 cup chopped green pepper
1/2 cup chopped onion
1 clove garlic, minced
1 tablespoon cooking oil
1 16-ounce can tomatoes, cut up
1 8-ounce can tomato sauce
1/2 cup dry white or red wine
3 tablespoons snipped parsley
1/4 teaspoon dried oregano, crushed
1/4 teaspoon dried basil, crushed
Dash of pepper
1 6 1/2-ounce can minced clams
1 4 1/2-ounce can shrimp, rinsed and drained

1. Make sure fish is thawed; cut into bite-size pieces.
2. Cook green pepper, onion and garlic in hot oil until tender.
3. Add tomatoes, tomato sauce, wine and next 4 ingredients; bring to a boil.
4. Reduce heat, cover and simmer 20 minutes.
5. Add fish, clams (with juices) and shrimp; boil and quickly reduce heat.
6. Cover and simmer 6 minutes; serve.

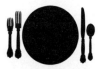

☑ Nutrition Information

Calories	260
Carbohydrates (grams)	14
Proteins (grams)	35
Cholesterol (milligrams)	113
Sodium (milligrams)	710
Fat (grams)	6.2
Saturated Fat (grams)	1.3

Wiener Schnitzel

SERVES 4

1 pound veal cutlets (1/4-inch thick)
2 tablespoons all-purpose flour
1 teaspoon minced fresh parsley
1/2 teaspoon pepper
1/4 teaspoon paprika
1/8 teaspoon ground cloves
Vegetable cooking spray
1 teaspoon vegetable oil, divided
1-1/2 teaspoons minced fresh parsley

---

1. *Trim veal of all fat*
2. *Using a meat mallet, pound down to 1/8 inch thickness.*
3. *Combine flour, parsley,pepper, paprika and cloves.*
4. *Dredge cutlets in flour mixture.*
5. *Coat a nonstick skillet with cooking spray and a 1/2 teaspoon oil. Place over medium-high heat and when hot add half of the cutlets. Brown well, about 3 minutes each side.*
6. *Remove from skillet and wipe skillet clean.*
7. *Repeat procedure with remaining cutlets and 1/2 teaspoon oil.*
8. *Sprinkle with parsley and serve.*

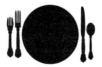

☑ *Nutrition Information*

Calories	154
Carbohydrates (grams)	3.1
Proteins (grams)	23.3
Cholesterol (milligrams)	94
Sodium (milligrams)	98
Fat (grams)	4.7
Saturated Fat (grams)	2.4

Chicken Jambalaya

SERVES 6
1 cup long-grain rice
1 large onion, chopped
1/2 cup chopped celery
1/2 cup chopped green pepper
2 cloves garlic, minced
2 tablespoons of diet margarine
1 16-ounce can tomatoes, cut up
1/2 of a 6-ounce can (1/3 cup) tomato paste
1/2 cup chopped smoked turkey sausage
1 teaspoon Creole seasoning
2 whole large chicken breasts (about 2 lbs. total),
skinned, boned, and cut into bite-size pieces
1/4 teaspoon bottled hot pepper sauce

1. *Cook rice; set aside.*
2. *In a large saucepan cook onion, celery, green pepper and garlic in diet margarine until tender.*
3. *Stir in tomatoes with liquid, tomato paste, turkey sausage and Creole seasoning. Bring to a boil then cover and simmer for 30 minutes.*
4. *Add chicken and hot pepper sauce; simmer about 15 minutes more.*
5. *Stir in rice and heat through, stirring occasionally.*

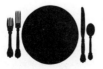

☑ *Nutrition Information*

Calories	252
Carbohydrates (grams)	20
Proteins (grams)	28
Cholesterol (milligrams)	73
Sodium (milligrams)	500
Fat (grams)	6.1
Saturated Fat (grams)	1.5

Italian-Rolled Steak

> **SERVES 8**
> 1/2 cup fresh breadcrumbs
> 1/2 cup minced fresh parsley
> 1/3 cup (1-1/3 ounces) grated fresh Parmesan cheese
> 3 tablespoons capers
> 2 tablespoons pine nuts, toasted
> 2 tablespoons fresh lemon juice
> 1 teaspoon olive oil • 4 garlic cloves, minced
> 1 (1-1/2-pound) lean flank steak
> Vegetable cooking spray
> 1-1/2 cups low-fat spaghetti sauce
> 1/2 cup dry red wine
> 8 cups hot cooked fettuccine (about 16 ozs.
> uncooked pasta)

1. Combine first 8 ingredients in a bowl and stir well; set aside.
2. Trim steak of all visible fat. Cut steak in half, horizontally through the center; DO NOT cut through other side of steak.
3. Open steak and lay flat; pound with a meat mallet to even out thickness.
4. Spread breadcrumb mixture over steak; leave a 1-inch margin around outside edges of steak.
5. Roll the steak, jelly-roll fashion, secure as you go with string.
6. Brown steak over medium-high heat in a large Dutch oven.
7. After all sides are browned, remove from pan and keep warm.
8. Add spaghetti sauce and wine to pan; bring to a boil and return steak to pan.
9. Cover, reduce heat and simmer 1 hour. Remove string from steak before cutting into 16 slices.
10. Serve 2 slices of steak over 1 cup pasta and 1/3 cup sauce.

☑ **Nutrition Information**

Calories	410
Carbohydrates (grams)	44
Proteins (grams)	24.9
Cholesterol (milligrams)	46
Sodium (milligrams)	531
Fat (grams)	14.2
Saturated Fat (grams)	5.2

Chicken Scaloppini

SERVES 4
1 lemon
4 skinless, boneless chicken breast halves (about 1 lb)
2 tablespoons flour
1/4 teaspoon salt
1/8 teaspoon freshly ground black pepper
3 teaspoons olive oil
1 garlic clove, crushed
1 green, 1 red and 1 yellow bell pepper, cut into
1/4-inch-wide strips
1/3 cup dry white wine
1/2 cup low-sodium chicken stock
2 teaspoons cornstarch
1 tablespoon finely chopped parsley

1. Cut lemon in half; squeeze 1 tablespoon juice from 1 half and slice the other half.
2. Cut chicken breasts in half, splitting them crosswise.
3. Flatten and sprinkle with flour, salt and pepper to coat.
4. Heat oil and garlic in nonstick pan until oil is hot. Discard garlic.
5. Add 1 layer of chicken to pan and saute about 1 minute each side. Remove to plate; keep warm and repeat procedure with remaining chicken.
6. Add peppers, wine and lemon juice to pan; cook, covered, 5 minutes over low heat.
7. Uncover, raise heat to high and cook 5 more minutes until sauce is reduced to 2 tablespoons.
8. Stir together stock and corn starch then stir into sauce; boil and cook 1 minute. Stir in parsley; pour over chicken; garnish with sliced lemon.

☑ **Nutrition Information**

Calories	228
Carbohydrates (grams)	5.8
Proteins (grams)	29.7
Cholesterol (milligrams)	70
Sodium (milligrams)	217
Fat (grams)	8
Saturated Fat (grams)	2

Pecan Creamed Chicken

SERVES 4
1/3 cup coarsely chopped pecans
2 tablespoons light margarine
4 large chicken breasts, skinless, boneless
4 tablespoons flour
1/4 teaspoon ground pepper
6 ounce cream cheese, nonfat
1 cup skim milk

1. In a nonstick pan, saute pecans in 1 tablespoon diet margarine.
2. Cut chicken breasts in half.
3. Combine flour and pepper in a bag; add chicken and shake to coat.
4. Add 1 tablespoon diet margarine to skillet; over medium-high heat brown chicken about 2 minutes each side.
5. Remove to serving dish.
6. Add nonfat cream cheese and skim milk to skillet; boil and whisk until cheese blends into a smooth sauce.
7. Add pecans to sauce; pour over chicken and serve.

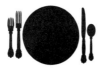

☑ Nutrition Information

Calories	357
Carbohydrates (grams)	18
Proteins (grams)	40
Cholesterol (milligrams)	93
Sodium (milligrams)	235
Fat (grams)	12.7
Saturated Fat (grams)	2.0

Tokyo Tuna Sandwich

SERVES 4
3/4 pound tuna fillet
1/4 cup reduced-sodium soy sauce
2 tablespoons lemon juice
2 tablespoons dry sherry
1 tablespoon grated ginger
2 teaspoons to 1 tablespoon freshly ground pepper
Vegetable cooking spray
1/2 teaspoon wasabi powder
1 teaspoon water
2 tablespoons fat free mayonnaise
4 (3/4-oz) slices reduced-calorie whole wheat
bread, toasted
1/2 cup alfalfa sprouts

1. *Place tuna in a shallow baking dish.*
2. *Combine soy sauce, lemon juice, sherry, and ginger in a small bowl. Pour mixture over tuna and marinate, covered, 1-2 hours in the refrigerator.*
3. *Remove tuna from marinade and discard marinade.*
4. *Sprinkle tuna with pepper.*
5. *Broil tuna 5 minutes each side then transfer to a bowl and flake.*
6. *Combine wasabi powder and water; add mayonnaise; stir well.*
7. *Spread mayonnaise mixture on toasted bread and divide tuna among prepared bread.*
8. *Top with alfalfa sprouts and serve.*

✓ **Nutrition Information**

Calories	216
Carbohydrates (grams)	14
Proteins (grams)	25
Cholesterol (milligrams)	35
Sodium (milligrams)	746
Fat (grams)	5.2
Saturated Fat (grams)	1.3

Jalapeno Chicken

SERVES 4
2 medium tomatoes, peeled and seeded
3 tablespoons cider vinegar
1 tablespoon plus 2 teaspoons dark molasses
1 tablespoon Dijon mustard
1 small jalapeno pepper, seeded and chopped
3 cloves garlic, pressed
1/4 teaspoon salt
4 (4-ounce) skinned, boned chicken breast halves

1. *Process Tomatoes in a blender until smooth.*
2. *Combine with next 6 ingredients in a casserole dish.*
3. *Cover and microwave on high for 5 minutes; set aside.*
4. *Place chicken in a baking dish; spoon tomato puree over chicken.*
5. *Cover and microwave on high 10-12 minutes or until chicken is done.*
6. *Let stand 3 minutes before serving.*

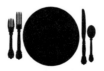

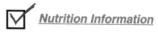 **Nutrition Information**

Calories	167
Carbohydrates (grams)	9.0
Proteins (grams)	26.9
Cholesterol (milligrams)	73
Sodium (milligrams)	337
Fat (grams)	3.0
Saturated Fat (grams)	0.9

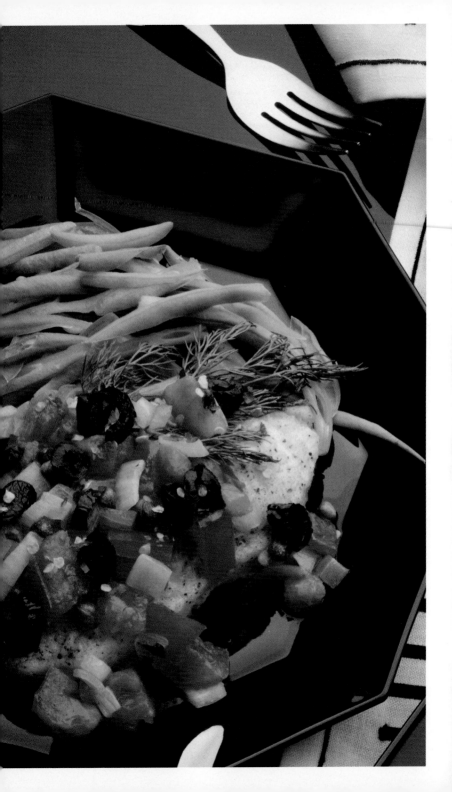

Swordfish Italiano

Heart-smart fish oils abound in this simple, delectable dish.

Photo Credits
Photography by Barney Taxel
Barney Taxel & Co.
216/431-2400

Recipe Credits
Swordfish Italiano, see page 63
Servings: 4

Island Grouper with Carambola Salsa

SERVES 6
2 medium carambola (starfruit), thinly sliced
1 cup fresh strawberries, hulled and sliced
1/2 cup finely chopped onion
1 tablespoon chopped jalapeno pepper
1 tablespoon minced fresh cilantro
1 teaspoon grated lime rind
1 tablespoon lime juice
1/4 teaspoon ground coriander
1/8 teaspoon ground red pepper
2 tablespoons lime juice
2 teaspoons reduced-calorie margarine, melted
6 (4-ounce) grouper fillets
Vegetable cooking spray

1. *Combine first 9 ingredients in a bowl; cover and chill 2 hours.*
2. *Combine lime juice and margarine; stir well.*
3. *Place fillets on a broiler rack coated with cooking spray; brush with lime mixture.*
4. *Broil until fish flakes easily when tested with a fork.*
5. *Spoon salsa over fillets and serve.*

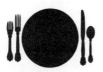

Nutrition Information

Calories	134
Carbohydrates (grams)	9.9
Proteins (grams)	21
Cholesterol (milligrams)	54
Sodium (milligrams)	79
Fat (grams)	1.2
Saturated Fat (grams)	0.3

Mexican Black Beans and Rice

SERVES 4
2 teaspoons olive oil
1 cup chopped onion
1/2 cup chopped green pepper
2 cups cooked long-grain rice (cooked
without salt or fat)
1/2 teaspoon ground cumin
1/4 teaspoon ground red pepper
1/8 teaspoon dried coriander
1 (15-ounce) can black beans, rinsed and drained
3/4 cup chopped tomato

1. In a nonstick skillet, heat oil until hot; add onion and green pepper and saute until tender.
2. Stir in rice, cumin, red pepper and coriander; saute 3 minutes.
3. Add beans and chopped tomato; saute until thoroughly heated; serve.

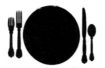

☑ *Nutrition Information*

Calories	246
Carbohydrates (grams)	47.4
Proteins (grams)	7.6
Cholesterol (milligrams)	0
Sodium (milligrams)	6
Fat (grams)	3.0
Saturated Fat (grams)	0.8

Shepherds Pie

SERVES 6

18 ounces lean ground beef
1 cup chopped onion
1 cup sliced steamed or microwaved carrots
1 cup sliced mushrooms
1 cup canned Ready Cut tomatoes
1-1/2 teaspoons Worcestershire sauce
1/2 teaspoon dried rosemary
2-1/2 tablespoons all-purpose flour
1 cup beef broth or bouillon
5 small potatoes
1/4 cup (4 tablespoons) diet margarine
1/4 cup non-fat milk, heated
1/4 cup chopped parsley
Salt and pepper to taste

1. Saute ground beef and onion in a non-stick skillet coated with cooking spray. Drain off fat.
2. Add carrots and next 4 ingredients; simmer 10 minutes.
3. Combine flour and beef broth; add to meat mixture and cook about 5 minutes or until mixture thickens.
4. Peel potatoes and cut in half. Boil potatoes about 15 minutes; drain and mash.
5. Add margarine and milk to potatoes. Add parsley and mix well.
6. Season with salt and pepper.
7. Place meat mixture in a casserole dish; cover with mashed potatoes.
8. Bake in preheated 450 oven for 20 minutes.

☑ **Nutrition Information**

Calories	261
Carbohydrates (grams)	22
Proteins (grams)	19
Cholesterol (milligrams)	53
Sodium (milligrams)	280
Fat (grams)	10.6
Saturated Fat (grams)	4.1

Crab-Stuffed Wontons

SERVES 4

1/3 pound fresh lump crab meat, drained
1/4 cup egg substitute
2 tablespoons minced green onions
1 clove garlic, minced • 1/2 teaspoon sesame oil
1/4 teaspoon dry mustard • 3 to 4 drops hot sauce
24 fresh or frozen wonton skins, thawed
1 egg white, lightly beaten • Oriental Tomato Sauce
Fresh cilantro sprigs (optional)
Oriental Tomato Sauce: Vegetable cooking spray
2 tablespoons chopped green onions
2 cloves garlic, minced
1-1/2 teaspoons peeled, minced ginger
1/4 cup canned low-sodium chicken broth, undiluted
1 (14-1/2 ounce) can no-salt-added whole
tomatoes, drained and chopped
1/8 teaspoon salt and dash of ground white pepper

1. Combine first 7 ingredients in a bowl; mix to blend.
2. Place 1 tablespoon crab meat mixture in center of 12 wonton skins. Brush edges of wonton skins with egg white; top with remaining 12 wonton skins. Press wonton edges together to seal.
3. Boil water in a large pot; add wontons and return to a boil.
4. Reduce heat and simmer 5 minutes.
5. Remove wontons and evenly distribute between 4 serving plates.
6. Top with oriental tomato sauce. For Sauce: Place a medium-size nonstick pan (coated with cooking spray) over medium-high heat; when pan is hot add green onions, garlic and ginger; saute 1 minute, stirring constantly; add chicken broth and cook 2 minutes; add remaining ingredients and cook 5 minutes more.

☑ **Nutrition Information**

Calories	90
Carbohydrates (grams)	6.7
Proteins (grams)	11.2
Cholesterol (milligrams)	29
Sodium (milligrams)	531
Fat (grams)	1.8
Saturated Fat (grams)	0.2

Grecian Sole Fillets

SERVES 8
Vegetable cooking spray
1/4 cup chopped onion
1/4 cup diced sweet red pepper
1 clove garlic, minced
1 (10-ounce) package frozen chopped spinach,
thawed and well drained
1/2 cup crumbled feta cheese
2 tablespoons sliced ripe olives
1 teaspoon grated lemon rind
1/2 teaspoon dried whole basil
1/4 teaspoon dried whole oregano
1/8 teaspoon ground white pepper
8 (4-ounce) sole fillets
1/4 teaspoon paprika

1. *Coat a nonstick pan with cooking spray; heat until hot.*
2. *Add onion, red pepper and garlic; saute about 3 minutes.*
3. *Remove from heat and combine with spinach, cheese and next 5 ingredients; stir well.*
4. *Place about 3 tablespoon spinach mixture onto each fillet and roll up jelly roll fashion.*
5. *Place a toothpick into center of each fillet to secure; season   with paprika.*
6. *Coat a baking dish with cooking spray; place rolls seam side down in baking dish.*
7. *Bake for 25 minutes, uncovered, in a 350 oven. Remove toothpicks before serving.*

☑ Nutrition Information

Calories	149
Carbohydrates (grams)	3.0
Proteins (grams)	24.1
Cholesterol (milligrams)	64
Sodium (milligrams)	268
Fat (grams)	4.3
Saturated Fat (grams)	2.7

French-Style Chicken Stew

SERVES 8
4 (4-oz) skinned, boned chicken breast halves
2 teaspoons olive oil
1 cup thinly sliced green onions
1/2 cup sliced onion
4 cloves garlic, minced
2 cups peeled, chopped tomato
1-1/2 cups canned no-salt-added chicken
broth, undiluted
1 cup Chablis or other dry white wine
1 bay leaf
1 teaspoon dried whole thyme
1/2 teaspoon fennel seeds, crushed
1/4 teaspoon salt
1/8 teaspoon saffron powder
Dash of ground red pepper
2-1/3 cups sliced new potatoes
Freshly ground pepper (optional)

1. Poach chicken in a large saucepan; simmer at least 15 minutes.
2. Drain chicken; set aside.
3. Heat olive oil in a Dutch oven; when hot add onions and garlic and saute. Shred chicken into small pieces.
4. Add tomatoes, chicken broth, wine and bay leaf to onion mixture; stir well. Add thyme and next 4 ingredients and stir well.
5. Boil; cover and simmer over low heat 20 minutes.
6. Add potatoes; cook another 30 minutes.
7. Discard bay leaf and serve.

Nutrition Information

Calories	137
Carbohydrates (grams)	11.6
Proteins (grams)	15.1
Cholesterol (milligrams)	35
Sodium (milligrams)	137
Fat (grams)	3.2
Saturated Fat (grams)	0.9

Balsamic Beef Stew

SERVES 9
1-1/2 pounds lean boneless round steak (1/2-inch thick)
Vegetable cooking spray
1 large onion, sliced
1 clove garlic, minced
3-1/4 cups water
1/2 cup balsamic vinegar
1 tablespoon chopped fresh oregano
1 teaspoon chopped fresh parsley
1 teaspoon chopped fresh basil
2 teaspoons beef-flavored bouillon granules
1/2 teaspoon cracked pepper
2 medium-size sweet red peppers, cut into 1-inch pieces
2 medium sweet yellow peppers, cut into 1-inch pieces
1 cup sliced fresh mushrooms
1/4 lb snow pea pods, trimmed and cut into 1-inch pieces

1. *Trim steak of all visible fat; cut into bite size pieces.*
2. *Coat Dutch oven with cooking spray and heat; When hot add steak and brown well on all sides.*
3. *Remove steak and pat dry; Wipe drippings from Dutch oven.*
4. *Coat Dutch oven with cooking spray again; when hot, saute onion and garlic.*
5. *Stir in steak, water and next 4 ingredients.*
6. *Add bouillon and pepper, stirring well.*
7. *Bring to a boil; reduce heat and simmer about 1-1/2 hours.*
8. *Add pepper and mushrooms; cover and cook 15 minutes.*
9. *Add snow peas; cover and cook 15 minutes more; serve.*

☑ Nutrition Information

Calories	145
Carbohydrates (grams)	6.2
Proteins (grams)	17.8
Cholesterol (milligrams)	47
Sodium (milligrams)	250
Fat (grams)	5.3
Saturated Fat (grams)	1.2

Pork Chops Diablo

SERVES 6
1/3 cup reduced-calorie catsup
2 teaspoons prepared horseradish
2 teaspoons reduced-sodium Worcestershire sauce
1 teaspoon prepared mustard
1/2 teaspoon garlic powder
1/2 teaspoon chili powder
1/8 teaspoon poultry seasoning
1/8 teaspoon pepper
6 (6-oz.) lean center-cut loin pork chops (1/2-inch thick)
Vegetable cooking spray
Fresh parsley sprigs

1. Combine first 8 ingredients in a bowl; stir well; set aside.
2. Trim chops of all visible fat.
3. Coat a nonstick pan with cooking spray and heat.
4. Add chops and brown well, about 3 minutes each side.
5. Pour mixture over chops and bring to a boil.
6. Reduce heat, cover and simmer 40-50 minutes.
7. Garnish with parsley and serve.

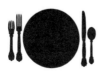

☑ Nutrition Information

Calories	215
Carbohydrates (grams)	1.9
Proteins (grams)	24.3
Cholesterol (milligrams)	77
Sodium (milligrams)	83
Fat (grams)	11.3
Saturated Fat (grams)	3.4

Sole Bonne Femme

SERVES 4
1-1/2 pounds sole fillets
Pepper
2 tablespoons minced shallots
2 tablespoons freshly chopped parsley
1 cup minced mushrooms
1/2 cup dry vermouth or wine
Juice of 1 lemon
1/4 teaspoon thyme
Sauce:
1/2 cup skim milk
1/2 cup bottled clam juice
1/8 teaspoon turmeric
2 tablespoons cold water
1 tablespoon cornstarch
White pepper to taste

1. Dry sole fillets and season both sides with pepper; set aside.
2. Combine remaining ingredients in a shallow baking dish.
3. Fold fillets crosswise, smooth side in, and arrange on top of vegetables. Heat dish on top of stove until liquid is just boiling.
4. Remove to a preheated 350 oven and bake, uncovered, for 10-12 minutes. Transfer fillets to a heated serving platter.
5. Drain mushroom mixture and add to fillets.
6. For sauce: Combine milk, clam juice and turmeric in a small saucepan; bring just to a boil; dissolve cornstarch in cold water; stir slowly into liquid until sauce returns to a boil; season with pepper.
7. Spoon prepared fish sauce over fillets and serve immediately.

☑ **Nutrition Information**

Calories	193
Carbohydrates (grams)	5
Proteins (grams)	30
Cholesterol (milligrams)	8
Sodium (milligrams)	142
Fat (grams)	1.9
Saturated Fat (grams)	0.5

Scotch Salmon

SERVES 4
4 (6-ounce) salmon steaks
1 onion, chopped
1 carrot, chopped
1 celery rib, chopped
2 tablespoons diet margarine
1 cup water
1/2 cup dry white wine
4 peppercorns, crushed
2 cloves
1 bay leaf

1. *In a nonstick skillet, saute onions, carrots, and celery over medium heat in diet margarine for 3 minutes.*
2. *Add remaining ingredients, except salmon.*
3. *Cover and simmer 5 minutes.*
4. *Place salmon steaks carefully into skillet.*
5. *Cover and simmer 8-10 minutes then serve.*

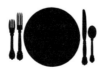

☑ Nutrition Information

Calories	208
Carbohydrates (grams)	2
Proteins (grams)	24
Cholesterol (milligrams)	31
Sodium (milligrams)	1112
Fat (grams)	8.6
Saturated Fat (grams)	1.7

Grilled Pork with Sweet and Tangy Cabbage

SERVES 8

1/2 cup canned no-salt-added beef broth, undiluted
1/4 cup unsweetened apple juice
1/4 cup chopped onion • 2 tablespoons cider vinegar
2 tablespoons low-sodium Worcestershire sauce
1 tablespoon chili powder • 2 cloves garlic, chopped
2 (1/2-pound) pork tenderloins
1/4 teaspoon freshly ground pepper • 1/8 teaspoon salt
Vegetable cooking spray
2 tablespoons no-salt-added tomato paste
2 (6-ounce) French bread baguettes
Sweet-and-Tangy Cabbage:
8 cups shredded cabbage
1 large purple onion, thinly sliced
1/2 cup water • 1/2 cup red wine vinegar
3 tablespoons sugar • 1/8 teaspoon salt
1/4 teaspoon freshly ground pepper

1. Combine first 7 ingredients in a large, heavy duty, zip lock freezer bag. Add Pork. Seal bag and shake well to coat pork.
2. Marinate in refrigerator for 8 hours, shaking bag occasionally.
3. Remove pork from bag, season with salt and pepper; reserve marinade. Grill over medium hot coals about 25 minutes; turn often.
4. In a saucepan boil reserved marinade; reduce heat and simmer 3 minutes; whisk in tomato paste and cook 3 minutes more.
5. Cut each baguette in quarters to make 8 sandwich rolls.
6. Slice pork into thin slices and divide evenly among sandwich rolls. Top with 2 tablespoons marinade and sweet and tangy cabbage.
7. Cabbage: in nonstick pan coated with cooking spray, combine first 7 ingredients; cover and cook until tender, about 55 minutes.

☑ **Nutrition Information**

Calories	256
Carbohydrates (grams)	37.5
Proteins (grams)	17.3
Cholesterol (milligrams)	40
Sodium (milligrams)	383
Fat (grams)	3.4
Saturated Fat (grams)	1.2

German Meatloaf with Ginger Glaze

SERVES 6
1 pound lean ground beef
3/4 cup soft breadcrumbs
1/4 cup egg substitute
1/2 cup finely chopped onion
1/2 cup finely chopped carrot
1/4 cup water
3 tablespoons gingersnap crumbs
2 tablespoons lemon juice
1/4 teaspoon salt
1/4 teaspoon pepper
Vegetable cooking spray
1 cup water
2 tablespoons lemon juice
1/4 cup gingersnap crumbs
2 tablespoons brown sugar
2 tablespoons raisins
1 teaspoon beef-flavored bouillon granules

1. Combine first 10 ingredients in a bowl; stir well to combine.
2. Place mixture int a loaf pan coated with cooking spray.
3. Bake 1 hour at 350; transfer to serving plate and keep warm.
4. Combine water, 2 tablespoons lemon juice, 1/4 cup gingersnap crumbs, brown sugar, raisins and bouillon in a saucepan; stir well.
5. Cook 10 minutes over medium heat, stirring occasionally.
6. Spoon over meatloaf and serve.

☑ Nutrition Information

Calories	305
Carbohydrates (grams)	25
Proteins (grams)	20
Cholesterol (milligrams)	47
Sodium (milligrams)	191
Fat (grams)	13.3
Saturated Fat (grams)	3.8

Lemon-Oregano Chicken

SERVES 4
2 large lemons
6 tablespoons fresh chopped parsley
3 teaspoons dried oregano
1-1/2 teaspoons ground pepper
4 large cloves garlic
1/2 teaspoon salt
4 chicken breast halves, skinless, boneless
2 tablespoons olive oil
1 cup plain nonfat yogurt

1. *Peel lemon; grate 3 teaspoons peel.*
2. *Cut lemons in half; cut 2 slices form 2 halves.*
3. *Squeeze 2 teaspoons juice from remaining lemons.*
4. *Place peels in bowl; add 4 tablespoons parsley, oregano and pepper.*
5. *Chop garlic and sprinkle with salt; add garlic to mixture in bowl.*
6. *Spoon 1 tablespoon seasoning mixture onto each chicken breast.*
7. *Drizzle olive oil over each breast.*
8. *Broil 12 minutes each side.*
9. *Garnish with lemon slices and serve with yogurt sauce.*
10. *For sauce: mix yogurt and 2 teaspoons lemon juice into remaining seasoning mixture.*

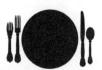

☑ Nutrition Information

Calories	237
Carbohydrates (grams)	4.5
Proteins (grams)	36
Cholesterol (milligrams)	93
Sodium (milligrams)	118
Fat (grams)	7
Saturated Fat (grams)	1.6

Baked Chicken in Aromatic Tomato Sauce

SERVES 6

2 tablespoons olive oil • 1/2 cup chicken broth
6 (6-ounce) chicken breasts cut into 12 pieces
3 cups chopped red onion • 6 whole all-spice
1 cinnamon stick • 1 teaspoon ground cumin
1 teaspoon paprika • 1/2 teaspoon ground nutmeg
1/2 teaspoon ground cloves • Pinch of cayenne pepper
1 28 ounce can whole Italian-style tomatoes, drained,
juices reserved, tomatoes chopped
1 cup water • 2 tablespoons red wine vinegar
2 tablespoons tomato paste
Pinch of sugar • 12 ounce spaghetti
Grated parmesan cheese

1. In a Dutch oven, heat oil and chicken broth.
2. Add chicken in batches and brown on all sides. Remove chicken.
3. Add onions to Dutch oven and saute about 5 minutes; add spices and stir 1 minute. Add tomatoes, tomato juices and water; stir.
4. Return chicken to Dutch oven; cover and simmer over low heat about 35 minutes or until chicken is very tender. Remove chicken to platter and cover.
5. Add 2 tablespoons vinegar, tomato paste and sugar to Dutch oven. Simmer until thickened, about 10 minutes; season with pepper and vinegar.
6. Remove from heat but cover to keep warm.
7. Cook pasta in a large pot; drain.
8. Transfer pasta to serving platter; top with chicken and sauce; sprinkle with cheese.

Nutrition Information

Calories	501
Carbohydrates (grams)	50
Proteins (grams)	40
Cholesterol (milligrams)	95
Sodium (milligrams)	549
Fat (grams)	14.6
Saturated Fat (grams)	3.7

Baja Lasagna

SERVES 6
1/4 cup chopped onion
2 (14-1/2 ounce) cans Ready Cut tomatoes
3 ounces canned diced green chiles
1 cup sliced mushrooms
2-2/3 cups drained, canned kidney beans
1 tablespoon chili powder
1 teaspoon cumin
8 corn tortillas, cut in 1-inch wide strips
8 ounces (2 cups) shredded low-fat Cheddar cheese
1 cup nonfat sour cream

1. *Coat nonstick skillet with cooking spray; add onions and saute 4 minutes.*
2. *Add tomatoes, chiles, mushrooms, beans, chili powder and cumin; simmer uncovered 10 minutes.*
3. *In a casserole dish, arrange 1/3 of the tortilla strips in a single layer. Pour 1/4 of the tomato mixture and 1/3 of the cheese over the tortilla layer.*
4. *Repeat layers of tortillas, tomato mixture and cheese twice.*
5. *End the last layer with sour cream, tomato mixture and cheese.*
6. *Bake in preheated 350 oven for 30 minutes*

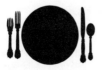

☑ Nutrition Information

Calories	307
Carbohydrates (grams)	41
Proteins (grams)	25
Cholesterol (milligrams)	60
Sodium (milligrams)	234
Fat (grams)	5.6
Saturated Fat (grams)	4.1

Oven-Fried Mustard Chicken

SERVES 6

1-1/2 tablespoons Dijon-style mustard
1 tablespoon lemon juice
3 large cloves garlic, finely minced
1/2 teaspoon crumbled dried rosemary
Freshly ground pepper
6 (4-ounce) chicken breasts, skinless and boneless
3 cups bran flakes cereal (or wheat or corn flakes)
6 tablespoons grated Parmesan cheese

1. Combine mustard, lemon juice, garlic, rosemary and pepper in a small bowl.
2. Coat chicken in mustard mixture.
3. In a zip top bag combine bran flakes and parmesan cheese; seal bag and crush bran flakes.
4. Add chicken breasts to bag and seal; shake well to coat.
5. Coat a baking dish with nonstick spray; place chicken in dish in a single layer and cover.
6. Bake in preheated 350 oven for 20 minutes.
7. Remove covering and bake another 20 minutes; serve.

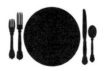

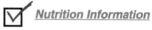
Nutrition Information

Calories	301
Carbohydrates (grams)	17
Proteins (grams)	40
Cholesterol (milligrams)	96
Sodium (milligrams)	1006
Fat (grams)	7.6
Saturated Fat (grams)	2.3

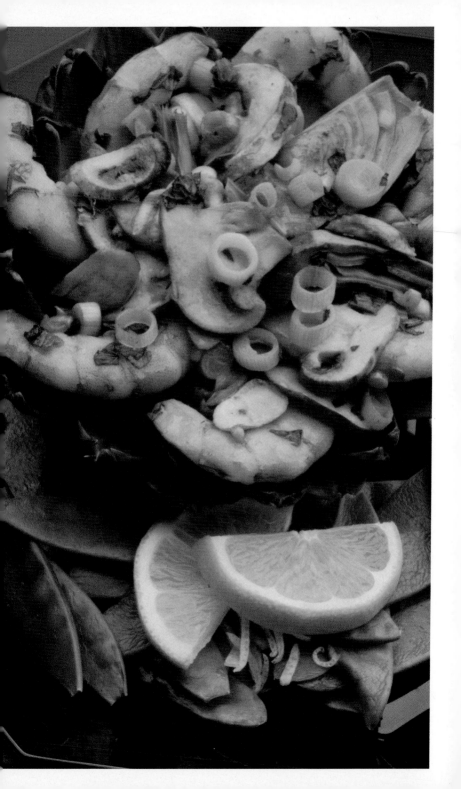

Artichoke Shrimp and Mushrooms

A tasty, gourmet combination to satisfy even the most discriminating palate.

Photo Credits
Photography by Barney Taxel
Barney Taxel & Co.
216/431-2400

Recipe Credits
Artichoke Shrimp and Mushrooms, see page 125
Servings: 4

Artichoke Shrimp and Mushrooms

SERVES 4
2 pounds unpeeled large fresh shrimp
Vegetable cooking spray
2 teaspoons olive oil
8 cloves garlic, coarsely chopped
2 tablespoon lime juice
1 cup sliced mushrooms
1 cup artichoke hearts, rinsed and cut in half

1. Peel and clean shrimp.
2. Coat a nonstick pan with cooking spray.
3. Add oil and garlic.
4. Over medium heat saute garlic 1 minute.
5. Add artichokes and mushrooms; saute 2-3 minutes (you may add a little water for moistness).
6. Add shrimp and cook about 4 minutes.
7. Add lime juice and cook an additional 3 minutes or until shrimp are done.

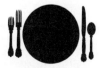

☑ *Nutrition Information*

Calories	223
Carbohydrates (grams)	6
Proteins (grams)	39
Cholesterol (milligrams)	348
Sodium (milligrams)	440
Fat (grams)	4.4
Saturated Fat (grams)	0.9

Broiled Split Fish with Pesto

SERVES 4
4 (6-ounce) flounder fillets
Pepper to taste
4 tablespoons prepared pesto sauce
2 cups cooked rice

1. *Season flounder with pepper.*
2. *Place under broiler 4 minutes each side or until fish flakes easily with fork.*
3. *Prepare pesto according to package directions; heat over low heat.*
4. *Place flounder over cooked rice.*
5. *Drizzle each fillet with 1 tablespoon pesto.*

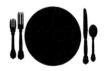

☑ Nutrition Information

Calories	311
Carbohydrates (grams)	30
Proteins (grams)	33
Cholesterol (milligrams)	91
Sodium (milligrams)	208
Fat (grams)	5
Saturated Fat (grams)	2

Italian-Style Frittata

SERVES 4
3 cups frozen egg substitute, thawed
1/8 teaspoon salt
1/8 teaspoon garlic powder
1/8 teaspoon pepper
3/4 cup chopped sweet red pepper
3/4 cup chopped green bell pepper
Nonstick cooking spray

1. *Coat a nonstick skillet with cooking spray.*
2. *Add red and green peppers and cook over low heat about 5 minutes.*
3. *Combine egg substitute, salt, garlic powder and pepper in a medium bowl; stir well.*
4. *Add mixture to skillet; turn heat to medium and cover.*
5. *Cook 8-10 minutes or until set.*

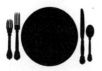

☑ Nutrition Information

Calories	181
Carbohydrates (grams)	6.7
Proteins (grams)	23
Cholesterol (milligrams)	2
Sodium (milligrams)	401
Fat (grams)	6.3
Saturated Fat (grams)	1.3

Asparagus Risotto with Mushrooms, Sundried Tomatoes

SERVES 6

1 tablespoon extra virgin olive oil
1 large onion, diced
1 large leek, halved and sliced thin
1 tablespoon finely minced garlic
2 cups uncooked rice, unrinsed
1/4 teaspoon freshly ground pepper
2 quarts low sodium vegetable broth (appr. 8 cups)
12 sun-dried tomatoes sliced thin
1 cup asparagus, sliced thin on the diagonal
1-1/2 cup sliced mushrooms
1/2 cup fresh basil, coarsely chopped

---

1. Over medium high heat, saute onion, leek and garlic in olive oil, about 3 minutes.
2. Add rice and pepper and saute 5 minutes.
3. In a separate pot, bring vegetable broth just to a boil then remove from heat.
4. Add 7 cups of broth and sundried tomatoes to rice mixture.
5. Reserve remaining 1 cup of broth.
6. Bring rice mixture to a boil; reduce heat and simmer for 15 minutes stirring often.
7. Steam asparagus, mushrooms, and basil about 5 minutes.
8. Add to rice mixture along with remaining 1 cup of broth.
9. Cook, stirring often until mixture is creamy and rice is done.

☑ Nutrition Information

Calories	186
Carbohydrates (grams)	35
Proteins (grams)	5.7
Cholesterol (milligrams)	0
Sodium (milligrams)	461
Fat (grams)	2.7
Saturated Fat (grams)	0.4

Grilled Jamaican Chicken

SERVES 4
4 skinned chicken breast halves
3 tablespoons lime juice
3 tablespoons lemon juice
3 tablespoons sweet vermouth
2 tablespoons Dijon mustard
1 jalapeno pepper, seeded and finely chopped
1 clove garlic, minced
1/4 teaspoon ground coriander
1/4 teaspoon dried oregano
1/4 teaspoon salt
cooking spray

1. *Place chicken in a dish and cover with next 10 ingredients.*
2. *Marinate in the refrigerator 8 hours, turning 2-3 times.*
3. *Remove chicken from marinade.*
4. *Pour marinade in a saucepan, boil then reduce heat and simmer 5 minutes.*
5. *Coat grill with cooking spray and grill chicken over medium coals 20 -25 minutes, turning and basting with marinade; serve.*

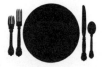

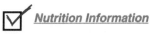

Nutrition Information

Calories	158
Carbohydrates (grams)	3.6
Proteins (grams)	25.9
Sodium (milligrams)	432
Fat (grams)	6.1
Saturated Fat (grams)	1.7

Crab Meat over Linguine

SERVES 4
8 ounces linguine, uncooked
1/2 pound fresh mushrooms, sliced
1/2 cup chopped green onion
1/2 cup chopped sweet red pepper
1/3 cup cream sherry
1 pound fresh crab meat, drained
1/4 cup chopped fresh parsley
2 teaspoons lemon juice

1. Cook linguine according to package directions (do not add salt or fat).
2. Drain and set aside.
3. Combine mushrooms, onions, pepper and sherry in a nonstick pan.
4. Cook over medium heat, stirring frequently.
5. Stir in crab meat, parsley and lemon juice; heat through.
6. Divide linguine among 4 serving plates; top with crab meat mixture.

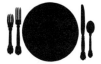

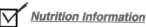

Nutrition Information

Calories	347
Carbohydrates (grams)	48.1
Proteins (grams)	30.4
Cholesterol (milligrams)	106
Sodium (milligrams)	309
Fat (grams)	3.1
Saturated Fat (grams)	0.4

Entrees

Honey Mustard Lamb Chops

SERVES 4
8 (3-ounce) lean lamb loin chops
2 cloves garlic, halved
1 tablespoon minced fresh rosemary
1/4 teaspoon freshly ground pepper
Nonstick cooking spray
1/4 cup honey
2 tablespoons stone ground mustard

1. *Trim chops of all visible fat.*
2. *Rub both sides of chops with cut side of garlic.*
3. *Season both sides of chops with rosemary and pepper.*
4. *Coat broiler pan with nonstick spray.*
5. *In a small bowl combine honey and mustard; set aside.*
6. *Place chops in broiler; broil one side 6 minutes then turn chops and spread with honey mustard sauce; broil additional 7 minutes; serve.*

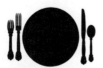

☑ Nutrition Information

Calories	259
Carbohydrates (grams)	18.7
Proteins (grams)	26.1
Cholesterol (milligrams)	81
Sodium (milligrams)	214
Fat (grams)	8.9
Saturated Fat (grams)	3.0

Apricot Glazed Ham

SERVES 4
1 (2 pounds) lean cooked, boneless ham,
cut into 8 slices
Nonstick cooking spray
1/3 cup reduced-calorie apricot spread
2 tablespoons unsweetened orange juice
2 tablespoons spicy hot mustard
1 teaspoon low sodium soy sauce
1/2 teaspoon peeled, grated ginger root

1. *Arrange ham slices in a baking dish coated with nonstick spray.*
2. *Combine apricot spread and remaining ingredients; spoon mixture evenly over ham slices.*
3. *Cover and bake at 325 for 15-20 minutes.*

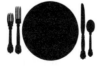

☑ *Nutrition Information*

Calories	158
Carbohydrates (grams)	10.5
Proteins (grams)	19.0
Cholesterol (milligrams)	48
Sodium (milligrams)	1198
Fat (grams)	4.7
Saturated Fat (grams)	1.4

Shrimp and Artichoke Quiche

SERVES 8
3 cups water
1 teaspoon liquid shrimp and crab boil seasoning
1 pound unpeeled medium size shrimp
nonstick cooking spray
1/3 cup Italian-seasoned breadcrumbs
3/4 cup frozen egg substitutes, thawed
1/4 cup all-purpose flour
1/2 teaspoon baking powder
1/4 teaspoon salt
1 (14-ounce) can artichoke hearts, drained and chopped
3/4 cup nonfat cottage cheese
1/2 cup shredded reduced fat Monterey Jack cheese
1/3 cup sliced green onions
1/4 cup shredded reduced-fat sharp cheddar cheese
1/2 teaspoon hot sauce

1. *Bring water and seasoning to a boil.*
2. *Add shrimp and cook 3-5 minutes.*
3. *Drain and rinse with cold water; peel and clean shrimp; chill.*
4. *Chop shrimp and set aside.*
5. *Coat a pie plate with cooking spray. Spread breadcrumbs around the sides and bottom of pie plate; set aside.*
6. *Stir together egg substitute, flour, baking powder and salt; add shrimp and artichoke hearts.*
7. *Add remaining ingredients.*
8. *Pour into pie plate and bake in 350 oven for 40 minutes or until set.*

☑ **Nutrition Information**

Calories	142
Carbohydrates (grams)	11.4
Proteins (grams)	18
Cholesterol (milligrams)	79
Sodium (milligrams)	520
Fat (grams)	2.8
Saturated Fat (grams)	1.4

Vietnamese-Style Wrapped Halibut

SERVES 4

4 (4-ounce) halibut fillets
2 tablespoons low sodium soy sauce
2 tablespoons dry sherry
1 tablespoon peeled, minced gingerroot
2 cloves garlic, minced
4 large Chinese cabbage leaves
1/4 cup sliced green onions
1 tablespoon minced fresh cilantro
1/4 teaspoon salt
1/8 teaspoon ground white pepper
2 tablespoons lemon juice

1. Combine soy sauce, sherry, gingerroot and garlic stirring well.
2. Place fillets in a baking dish. Pour marinade over fillets and cover. Refrigerate for 30 minutes.
3. Cook cabbage in boiling water for 30 seconds; Rinse under cold water; set aside.
4. Combine onion, cilantro, salt, and white pepper; stir well.
5. Remove fillets from marinade and discard marinade.
6. Drain cabbage leaves well.
7. Place one fillet at the base of cabbage leaf; spoon 1/4 of the onion mixture over fillet.
8. Fold sides of cabbage leaf over fillet as if you were wrapping a package. Repeat with remaining fillets.
9. Steam fillet over boiling water (covered) for 10-12 minutes.
10. Brush with lemon juice and serve.

☑ Nutrition Information

Calories	144
Carbohydrates (grams)	3.0
Proteins (grams)	24.6
Cholesterol (milligrams)	53
Sodium (milligrams)	339
Fat (grams)	2.7
Saturated Fat (grams)	0.4

Mahi-Mahi with Ginger and Lime

SERVES 6
2 (12-ounce) mahi-mahi fillets
1/4 cup lime juice
1 tablespoon honey
1 clove garlic, minced
1 (1/8-inch-thick) slice peeled ginger root
Nonstick cooking spray

1. *Cut each fillet into 3 equal pieces.*
2. *Place in a baking dish.*
3. *Stir together lime juice and next three ingredients; pour over fish.*
4. *Cover and marinate 1 hour.*
5. *Coat grill with cooking spray.*
6. *Remove fish from marinade; reserve marinade but discard ginger root.*
7. *Grill fish over medium hot coals 8 minutes each side, basting frequently with marinade.*

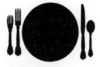

☑ Nutrition Information

Calories	109
Carbohydrates (grams)	4.1
Proteins (grams)	20.3
Cholesterol (milligrams)	49
Sodium (milligrams)	70
Fat (grams)	0.9
Saturated Fat (grams)	0.2

Red Snapper Veracruz

SERVES 4

4 (4-ounce) red snapper fillets (3/4-inch-thick)
Vegetable cooking spray
1-1/2 tablespoon fresh lime juice
1 medium onion, thinly sliced
3 cloves garlic, minced
2-1/2 cups peeled, chopped plum tomato
2 tablespoons chopped fresh cilantro
2 teaspoons seeded, minced serrano chile pepper
1/4 teaspoon salt
1/3 cup sliced ripe olives

1. Coat a baking dish with cooking spray.
2. Place fillets in dish; brush with lime juice; set aside.
3. In a nonstick skillet coated with cooking spray, saute onion and garlic about 3 minutes.
4. Stir in tomato and next 3 ingredients; cook 5 minutes.
5. Stir in olives.
6. Spoon mixture over fillets.
7. Cover and bake at 400 for 25 minutes.

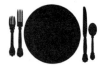

☑ Nutrition Information

Calories	173
Carbohydrates (grams)	10.9
Proteins (grams)	25.1
Cholesterol (milligrams)	42
Sodium (milligrams)	303
Fat (grams)	3.4
Saturated Fat (grams)	0.6

Spaghetti and Chickpea Sauce

SERVES 4
Nonstick cooking spray
2 teaspoons vegetable oil
1 medium onion, coarsely chopped
1 medium-size green pepper, chopped
2 cloves garlic, minced
1 tablespoon chopped fresh parsley
1 (15-ounce) can chick peas, drained
2 (8-ounce) cans no-salt-added tomato sauce
1/2 teaspoon dried whole oregano
1/4 teaspoon dried whole basil
1/4 teaspoon pepper
2 cups cooked spaghetti (cooked without salt/fat)
1/2 cup fine shred reduced-fat sharp cheddar cheese
1-1/2 tablespoon grated parmesan cheese

1. *In a large nonstick skillet coated with cooking spray, heat oil until hot.*
2. *Add onion, green pepper, garlic and parsley and saute 4 minutes.*
3. *Add chickpeas and next 4 ingredients; stir well.*
4. *Bring to a boil, stirring occasionally.*
5. *Reduce heat, cover and simmer about 30 minutes.*
6. *Top spaghetti with sauce, sprinkle with cheeses and serve.*

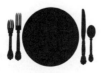

☑ *Nutrition Information*

Calories	438
Carbohydrates (grams)	72.4
Proteins (grams)	19.2
Cholesterol (milligrams)	11
Sodium (milligrams)	294
Fat (grams)	8.4
Saturated Fat (grams)	2.7

Lentil and Pasta Bake

SERVES 6

1 cup elbow macaroni, uncooked
3/4 cup dried lentils
3/4 cup chopped onion
1 medium carrot, finely chopped
1 clove garlic, minced
1-3/4 cup water
1 (8-ounce) can no salt added tomato sauce
2 tablespoons chopped fresh parsley
1/4 teaspoon ground cinnamon
1 tablespoon margarine
1-1/2 tablespoon all-purpose flour
1 cup skim milk
1/4 cup grated parmesan cheese
1/4 teaspoon salt
1/4 cup frozen egg substitute, thawed
Nonstick cooking spray

1. Cook macaroni using package directions (do not add salt or fat).
2. Combine lentils and next 4 ingredients in a saucepan; boil.
3. Reduce heat; cover and simmer about 30 minutes.
4. Stir in tomato sauce, parsley and cinnamon; set aside.
5. Melt margarine in a saucepan over medium heat; add flour and stir until smooth. Add milk slowly; cook stirring constantly until thickened. Add cheese and salt; stir until cheese melts.
6. Let mixture cool then add egg substitute.
7. In a baking dish coated with cooking spray layer 1/2 the macaroni mixture and 1/2 the lentil mixture. Repeat layers.
8. Top with cheese mixture. Bake, uncovered, in a 350 oven for 45 minutes.

☑ **Nutrition Information**

Calories	240
Carbohydrates (grams)	38.3
Proteins (grams)	14.1
Cholesterol (milligrams)	3
Sodium (milligrams)	235
Fat (grams)	3.7
Saturated Fat (grams)	1.2

Beef au Poivre

SERVES 12
1 (3-pound) beef tenderloin, trimmed of excess fat
3 tablespoons reduced calorie margarine, divided
1/2 teaspoon whole wheat peppercorn, coarsely crushed
1/2 teaspoon whole green peppercorn, coarsely crushed
1/2 teaspoon whole black peppercorn, coarsely crushed
Nonstick cooking spray
12 small round red potatoes
3 tablespoons water
2 tablespoons minced fresh chives
1 teaspoon coarsely ground pepper
1/2 teaspoon salt

1. *Combine 1-1/2 teaspoon margarine and all peppercorns in a small bowl; stir well. Rub mixture over entire surface of tenderloin.*
2. *Place tenderloin in a roasting pan well coated with cooking spray.*
3. *Combine remaining margarine, water, chives, pepper and salt in a bowl; stir well.*
4. *Cut potatoes into 1/4 inch slices; arrange potatoes around tenderloin. Brush potatoes with half of margarine mixture.*
5. *Bake at 400 for 20 minutes.*
6. *Reduce heat to 375 and bake and additional 35 minutes.*
7. *Remove tenderloin from roasting pan and set aside.*
8. *Brush potatoes with remaining margarine mixture; bake an additional 15 minutes.*
9. *Slice tenderloin diagonally across grain and arrange potatoes around tenderloin.*

☑ Nutrition Information

Calories	270
Carbohydrates (grams)	19.1
Proteins (grams)	25.9
Cholesterol (milligrams)	69
Sodium (milligrams)	172
Fat (grams)	8.8
Saturated Fat (grams)	3.2

Orange Steak Mandarin

SERVES 6
1 (1-1/2 pound) lean boneless sirloin steak
1 cup unsweetened orange juice
3 tablespoons lemon juice
1 teaspoon hot sauce
6 green onions, cut into 2-inch pieces
Nonstick cooking spray
1 tablespoon cornstarch
1/2 teaspoon salt
1 (11-oz) can mandarin oranges in heavy syrup, drained
4-1/2 cups cooked long-grain rice
(cook without salt or fat)

1. Trim steak of all visible fat
2. Place steak in heavy duty ziplock bag.
3. Mix together orange juice and next 3 ingredients.
4. Pour over steak; seal bag and shake to coat steak.
5. Marinate in refrigerator 3 hours, turning bag occasionally.
6. Remove steak from marinade; strain marinade and reserve green onions. Set onions and marinade aside.
7. Coat broiler rack with nonstick spray and broil steak 10-12 minutes. Turn steak and top with green onions; broil additional 10 minutes.
8. Slice steak diagonally into thin slices; set meat and onions aside.
9. In a small saucepan combine marinade, cornstarch and salt.
10. Boil over medium heat, stirring constantly.
11. In a bowl toss together steak, green onions, marinade mixture and oranges.
12. Spoon cooked rice onto serving platter; top with steak mixture.

☑ Nutrition Information

Calories	402
Carbohydrates (grams)	47.9
Proteins (grams)	31.5
Cholesterol (milligrams)	82
Sodium (milligrams)	266
Fat (grams)	8.3
Saturated Fat (grams)	3.3

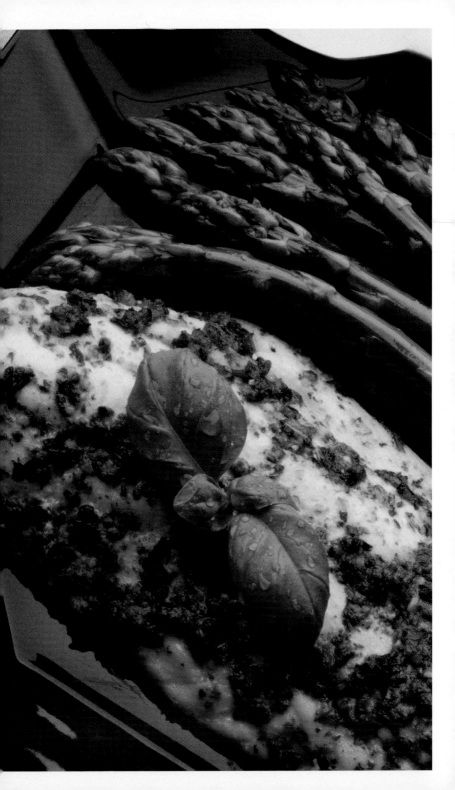

Broiled Split Fish with Pesto
Presto! Pesto turns this ordinary fish into a magical main course.

Photo Credits
Photography by Barney Taxel
Barney Taxel & Co.
216/431-2400

Recipe Credits
Broiled Split Fish with Pesto, see page 126
Servings: 4

Beef Burgundy

SERVES 6
1 (1-1/2 pound) lean boneless sirloin steak
Nonstick cooking spray
1 large onion, sliced and separated into rings
1/2 teaspoon salt
1/2 teaspoon dried whole oregano
1/2 teaspoon pepper
1/4 teaspoon garlic powder
1/4 teaspoon dried whole thyme
2 bay leaves
1 (13-3/4 ounce) can no salt added beef broth, undiluted
1-1/4 cup burgundy or other dry red wine
1-1/2 cup sliced fresh mushrooms
3 tablespoons cornstarch • 1/2 cup water
1/4 teaspoon browning-and-seasoning sauce
6 cups cooked medium egg noodles
(cooked without salt or fat)

1. Trim steak of all visible fat. Slice steak diagonally across grain into 1/4 inch strips.
2. Coat a Dutch oven with cooking spray and heat over medium heat until hot. Add steak and brown well.
3. Add onions and next 8 ingredients; stir well.
4. Bring to a boil then reduce heat, cover and simmer 20 minutes.
5. Add mushrooms, cover and simmer 5 minutes more.
6. Combine cornstarch, water and browning-and-seasoning sauce.
7. Add to steak mixture, stirring constantly.
8. Bring mixture to a boil; boil 1 minute to thicken, stirring constantly. Remove bayleaf.
9. Spoon mixture over noodles and serve.

Nutrition Information

Calories	409
Carbohydrates (grams)	48.3
Proteins (grams)	32.7
Cholesterol (milligrams)	122
Sodium (milligrams)	281
Fat (grams)	8.3
Saturated Fat (grams)	2.6

Classic Pot Roast

SERVES 12
1 (3 pound) beef eye-of-round roast
2 cloves garlic, thinly sliced
1/4 cup all-purpose flour
1/2 teaspoon salt
1/2 teaspoon coarsely ground pepper
Nonstick cooking spray
1 medium onion, sliced
1 bay leaf
1 cup burgundy or other red wine
1 (8-ounce) can no salt added tomato sauce
1 tablespoon brown sugar
1 teaspoon dried whole oregano
1 teaspoon prepared horseradish
1 teaspoon prepared mustard

1. *Trim roast of all visible fat.*
2. *Combine flour, salt and pepper. Dredge roast in flour mixture.*
3. *Cut 1 inch slits in roast and insert a garlic slice into each slit.*
4. *Coat a Dutch oven with cooking spray; place over medium-high heat. When hot add roast and brown on all sides.*
5. *Add onion and bayleaf.*
6. *Combine wine and next 5 ingredients; stir well. Pour over roast.*
7. *Bring to a boil; cover.*
8. *Reduce heat and simmer 1-2 hours until roast is tender.*
9. *Place roast and onion on a serving platter; top with remaining sauce.*

Nutrition Information

Calories	175
Carbohydrates (grams)	5.8
Proteins (grams)	25.4
Cholesterol (milligrams)	61
Sodium (milligrams)	169
Fat (grams)	5
Saturated Fat (grams)	1.8

Veal Piccata

SERVES 4
1 pound veal cutlets (1/4 inch thick)
1/4 cup all-purpose flour
Nonstick cooking spray
1 teaspoon olive oil
1/2 cup dry sherry
1/4 cup lemon juice
2 tablespoons capers

1. *Trim cutlets of all visible fat.*
2. *Dredge cutlets in flour.*
3. *Heat oil in a nonstick skillet coated with cooking spray.*
4. *Brown veal in skillet over medium-high heat, about 3-4 minutes each side.*
5. *Remove veal to serving platter; keep warm.*
6. *Wipe drippings from skillet.*
7. *Add sherry, lemon juice and capers to skillet; stir well.*
8. *Cook over medium-high heat until mixture is reduced by half, stirring constantly.*
9. *Pour over veal and serve.*

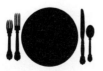

☑ **Nutrition Information**

Calories	178
Carbohydrates (grams)	8.7
Proteins (grams)	24
Cholesterol (milligrams)	94
Sodium (milligrams)	435
Fat (grams)	4.6
Saturated Fat (grams)	1.1

Veal in Green Peppercorn Sauce

SERVES 4
1 pound veal cutlets (1/4 inch thick)
Nonstick cooking spray
1-1/2 canned no salt added beef broth, undiluted
1/2 cup burgundy or other dry red wine
2 large cloves garlic crushed
2 bay leaves
1-1/2 tblspn. green peppercorns, drained and divided
1/2 teaspoon salt
1 tablespoon plus 1 teaspoon cornstarch
2 tablespoons water

1. Trim cutlets of all visible fat. Heat a nonstick skillet coated with cooking spray over medium-high heat.
2. When hot add veal and brown about 3 minutes each side.
3. Remove veal; wipe drippings from skillet.
4. Add broth and next 5 ingredients to skillet; add veal and bring to a boil. Cover, reduce heat and simmer 20 minutes.
5. Remove veal and set aside. Discard bay leaves.
6. Combine cornstarch and water stirring well.
7. Add to broth mixture and stir constantly until thickened.
8. Return veal to skillet and heat through; serve.

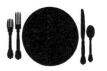

☑ Nutrition Information

Calories	194
Carbohydrates (grams)	4.2
Proteins (grams)	27.7
Cholesterol (milligrams)	100
Sodium (milligrams)	375
Fat (grams)	5.8
Saturated Fat (grams)	1.6

Bourbon-Marinated Veal with Onion Relish

SERVES 12
1 (3 pound) boneless veal roast
1 large clove garlic, halved
2/3 cup bourbon • 1/4 cup water
1/2 teaspoon hot sauce
3/4 teaspoon pepper, divided • 1/2 teaspoon salt
Nonstick cooking spray
Onion relish:
3 medium onions, quartered and thinly sliced
1-1/2 tablespoon brown sugar
1 tablespoon chopped fresh thyme
3 tablespoons white wine vinegar
1/2 teaspoon pepper

1. Trim roast of all visible fat; rub with garlic.
2. Place roast in a heavy duty ziplock bag.
3. Mix together bourbon, water, hot sauce and 1/2 teaspoon pepper; pour over veal roast. Seal bag and shake well to coat.
4. Marinate in refrigerator about 8 hours, turning occasionally.
5. Coat a roasting pan with cooking spray.
6. Remove roast from marinade and discard marinade.
7. Season roast with remaining 1/4 teaspoon pepper and salt.
8. Place in roasting pan, cover and bake in a 325 oven for 1-1/2 hours. Uncover and bake an additional 1 hour.
9. Let stand 10 minutes before slicing into 1/4 inch slices. Serve with onion relish.
10. Relish: heat a nonstick skillet coated with cooking spray over medium heat; when hot add onion; cover and simmer over low heat 2 hours. Add brown sugar, thyme, vinegar and pepper. Cook uncovered, stirring often 5-6 minutes.

☑ **Nutrition Information**

Calories	180
Carbohydrates (grams)	5.6
Proteins (grams)	25.5
Cholesterol (milligrams)	92
Sodium (milligrams)	268
Fat (grams)	5.3
Saturated Fat (grams)	1.5

Sicilian Veal Chops

SERVES 4
4 (6-ounce) lean veal loin chops
3/4 teaspoon dried Italian seasoning
1/8 teaspoon pepper
Nonstick cooking spray
1/4 cup water
1/4 cup Chablis or other dry white wine
1/2 teaspoon chicken flavored bouillon granules
1 clove garlic, crushed
1 small onion, thinly sliced
2 cups sliced fresh mushrooms
1/2 teaspoon dried whole rosemary, crushed
1 tablespoon chopped fresh parsley

1. Trim chops of all visible fat.
2. Season with italian seasoning and pepper.
3. Heat a nonstick skillet coated with cooking spray over medium-high heat.
4. When hot add chops and brown, about 4 minutes each side.
5. Remove from skillet and set aside.
6. Boil water and next three ingredients in skillet; reduce heat and simmer 2 minutes.
7. Place onion in a baking dish coated with cooking spray.
8. Place chops over onion. Pour wine mixture over chops; top with mushrooms and rosemary.
9. Cover and bake at 350 for 30-35 minutes. Sprinkle with parsley and serve.

☑ **Nutrition Information**

Calories	160
Carbohydrates (grams)	5.4
Proteins (grams)	24.2
Cholesterol (milligrams)	91
Sodium (milligrams)	211
Fat (grams)	4.4
Saturated Fat (grams)	1.2

Spicy Chicken Bake

SERVES 4
Nonstick cooking spray
1 teaspoon vegetable oil
4 (4-ounce) skinned, boned chicken breast halves,
cut into 1/2 inch strips
1 cup frozen whole kernel corn, thawed and drained
1/2 cup thinly sliced onions
1/3 cup chopped green peppers
1/2 cup no salt added tomato sauce
2-1/2 tablespoon reduced calorie chili sauce
2 tablespoons water
1-1/2 teaspoon minced fresh cilantro
1 teaspoon chili powder
1 teaspoon finely chopped jalapeno pepper
1/2 cup reduced fat Monterey Jack cheese, shredded

1. *Heat oil over medium-high heat in a nonstick skillet coated with cooking spray.*
2. *Add chicken and lightly brown, about 5 minutes.*
3. *Drain and pat dry; wipe drippings from skillet.*
4. *Combine chicken, corn and next 8 ingredients in a bowl; stir well.*
5. *Transfer mixture to a casserole dish coated with cooking spray.*
6. *Cover and bake at 350 for 30-35 minutes. Uncover, sprinkle with cheese and bake an additional 5 minutes.*

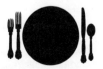

✓ Nutrition Information

Calories	265
Carbohydrates (grams)	16.4
Proteins (grams)	32.7
Cholesterol (milligrams)	82
Sodium (milligrams)	177
Fat (grams)	7.7
Saturated Fat (grams)	2.8

Turkey Milanese

SERVES 4
1/4 cup frozen egg substitute, thawed
2 teaspoons vegetable oil
1/2 cup fine, dry breadcrumbs
2 tablespoons grated parmesan cheese
3/4 teaspoon dried Italian seasoning
1/4 teaspoon garlic powder
1 pound turkey breast cutlets
Nonstick cooking spray
1/2 cup commercial Marinara sauce

1. Stir together egg substitute and oil.
2. Combine breadcrumbs and next 3 ingredients in a shallow dish.
3. Dip turkey into egg substitute mixture then dredge in breadcrumb mixture.
4. Coat a baking sheet with cooking spray.
5. Place turkey cutlets on baking sheet and spray lightly with cooking spray.
6. Bake at 350 for 20-25 minutes.
7. Heat marinara sauce until warm and pour over turkey cutlets.

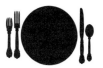

☑ Nutrition Information

Calories	248
Carbohydrates (grams)	13.4
Proteins (grams)	31.4
Cholesterol (milligrams)	71
Sodium (milligrams)	448
Fat (grams)	7.0
Saturated Fat (grams)	1.9

Rosemary Turkey

SERVES 6
3 (1/2 pound) turkey tenderloins
1-1/2 tablespoon finely chopped fresh rosemary
1 table spoon olive oil
1 large clove garlic, minced
1/4 teaspoon coarsely ground black pepper
1/4 teaspoon salt
Nonstick cooking spray
3 tablespoons dry vermouth
2 tablespoons water
1 teaspoon cornstarch

1. *Trim turkey of all visible fat.*
2. *Combine rosemary and next 4 ingredients.*
3. *Rub mixture on both sides of turkey.*
4. *Heat a nonstick skillet coated with cooking spray over medium-high heat.*
5. *When hot cook turkey about 7-8 minutes each side.*
6. *Slice turkey into thin slices and keep warm.*
7. *Combine vermouth, water and cornstarch; stir well.*
8. *Add to skillet; boil then reduce heat and simmer until thickened, stirring constantly.*
9. *Pour over turkey slices and serve.*

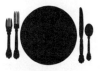

☑ Nutrition Information

Calories	332
Carbohydrates (grams)	1.6
Proteins (grams)	62.3
Cholesterol (milligrams)	159
Sodium (milligrams)	265
Fat (grams)	6.5
Saturated Fat (grams)	1.6

Japanese-Style Turkey

SERVES 6
3/4 cup rice wine
1/2 cup Chablis
3 tablespoons brown sugar
3 tablespoons low sodium soy sauce
1-1/2 pounds turkey tenderloins, cut into 1-inch cubes
1 large sweet red pepper, cut into 1-inch pieces
1 large green pepper, cut into 1-inch pieces
Nonstick cooking spray

1. *Combine first 4 ingredients in a saucepan; boil then reduce heat and simmer 5 minutes.*
2. *Place turkey in a heavy duty ziplock bag.*
3. *When wine mixture is cool add to bag.*
4. *Seal bag and shake to coat turkey well.*
5. *Marinate in refrigerator 6-8 hours, turning bag occasionally.*
6. *Reserve marinade.*
7. *Place turkey and pepper pieces alternately on skewers.*
8. *Coat grill with cooking spray.*
9. *Grill turkey kebabs over medium hot coals, basting with marinade frequently, about 7-8 minutes.*

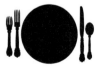

Nutrition Information

Calories	172
Carbohydrates (grams)	10
Proteins (grams)	24.4
Cholesterol (milligrams)	55
Sodium (milligrams)	254
Fat (grams)	3
Saturated Fat (grams)	0.9

Stuffed Cabbage

SERVES 6
6 large cabbage leaves
1/2 pound freshly ground turkey
1/2 pound lean ground pork
1 cup cooked brown rice
1/2 cup chopped onion
1 teaspoon dried Italian seasoning
1/8 teaspoon garlic powder
1/8 teaspoon salt
1/8 teaspoon pepper
2 (8-ounce) cans no salt added tomato sauce
1 teaspoon dried Italian seasoning
1/2 teaspoon salt
1/2 teaspoon pepper
1/4 teaspoon garlic powder

1. Boil water; cook cabbage leaves in boiling water about 6 minutes; drain and set aside.
2. In a bowl combine ground turkey and next 7 ingredients.
3. Place approximately 1/2 cup turkey mixture in center of each cabbage leave. Fold end of cabbage leaf over and roll up.
4. Combine tomato sauce, italian seasoning, salt, pepper and garlic powder; stir well.
5. Place cabbage rolls, seam side down, in a baking dish.
6. Pour sauce over cabbage rolls. Cover and bake at 350 for 1 hour.

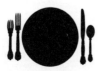

☑ *Nutrition Information*

Calories	190
Carbohydrates (grams)	18.7
Proteins (grams)	18.7
Cholesterol (milligrams)	47
Sodium (milligrams)	325
Fat (grams)	4.4
Saturated Fat (grams)	1.4

Monte Cristo Sandwich

SERVES 4
1/2 cup skim milk
1 egg lightly beaten
2 egg whites, lightly beaten
1/3 cup nonfat sour cream
3 tablespoons low sugar strawberry jam
4 (1-ounce) slices reduced fat swiss cheese
4 (1-ounce) slices roast turkey breast
8 (1-ounce) slices french bread
2/3 cup finely crushed shredded whole
wheat cereal biscuits

1. Combine milk, egg and egg whites in a shallow bowl.
2. In a separate bowl combine sour cream and strawberry jam.
3. Make 4 sandwiches consisting of 1 slice turkey and 1 slice cheese.
4. Dip sandwiches into egg mixture.
5. Place each sandwich on a baking sheet coated with cooking spray.
6. Sprinkle sandwiches with cereal.
7. Bake at 400 for 3 minutes; turn sandwiches and bake an additional 5 minutes or until crisp.
8. Serve with strawberry/sour cream mixture.

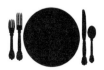

☑ Nutrition Information

Calories	411
Carbohydrates (grams)	50
Proteins (grams)	30.2
Cholesterol (milligrams)	95
Sodium (milligrams)	454
Fat (grams)	8.8
Saturated Fat (grams)	3.9

4
Desserts

Caribbean Melon Balls

SERVES 6
1/4 cup unsweetened orange juice
1 tablespoon sugar
2 tablespoons midori liquor
1 tablespoon lemon juice
1 teaspoon grated fresh ginger
1 cup each - cantaloupe, honeydew, watermelon balls
2 tablespoons chopped fresh mint

1. *Combine first 5 ingredients in a microwave-safe dish.*
2. *Cover and vent.*
3. *Heat on high until sugar dissolves (1-2 minutes).*
4. *In a large bowl, combine melon and mint.*
5. *Pour juice over melon.*
6. *Chill at least 2 hours.*

☑ Nutrition Information

Calories	49
Carbohydrates (grams)	10.9
Proteins (grams)	0.7
Cholesterol (milligrams)	0
Sodium (milligrams)	7
Fat (grams)	0.2
Saturated Fat (grams)	0

Baked Apples with Cream

SERVES 4
2 tablespoons light margarine
1/2 teaspoon ground cinnamon
4 tablespoons flour
2 teaspoons water
2-4 packets sugar substitute
4 medium size green apples
4 teaspoons fresh lemon juice
4 tablespoons water
1 cup light whipped topping

1. *In a bowl combine margarine, sugar substitute, cinnamon and flour until smooth.*
2. *Mix in water.*
3. *Peel and core apples.*
4. *Place 1 teaspoon lemon juice and 1 tablespoon water in each of 4 serving cups.*
5. *Roll apples in lemon juice mixture to coat.*
6. *Place 1 teaspoon margarine mixture in each apple.*
7. *Press remaining margarine mixture over tops of apples.*
8. *Bake in the center of a preheated 375 oven for 40 minutes.*
9. *Serve warm with a dollop of whipped cream.*

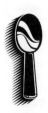

✓ Nutrition Information

Calories	246
Carbohydrates (grams)	41
Proteins (grams)	2
Cholesterol (milligrams)	0
Sodium (milligrams)	87
Fat (grams)	8.2
Saturated Fat (grams)	4.7

Bananas in Orange Sauce

SERVES 4

2 tablespoons diet margarine
4 tablespoons light brown sugar
1/2 teaspoon ground cardamom
1/2 teaspoon grated orange peel
1/2 cup strained, fresh orange juice
4 teaspoon fresh lemon juice
4 small ripe bananas
1/3 cup nonfat sour cream

1. *Over medium-high heat boil all ingredients except bananas and sour cream.*
2. *Heat until mixture looks syrupy and is reduced to about 2/3 cup (about 4 minutes).*
3. *Peel bananas and remove strings.*
4. *Cut in half lengthwise and crosswise.*
5. *Add to sauce, cut side up, cook 1 minute basting with sauce.*
6. *Turn bananas over and cook until soft (about 1 minute more).*
7. *Remove bananas to serving plate; top with sauce and a dollop of sour cream.*

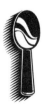

☑ *Nutrition Information*

Calories	268
Carbohydrates (grams)	50
Proteins (grams)	4.8
Cholesterol (milligrams)	0
Sodium (milligrams)	141
Fat (grams)	6.7
Saturated Fat (grams)	3.3

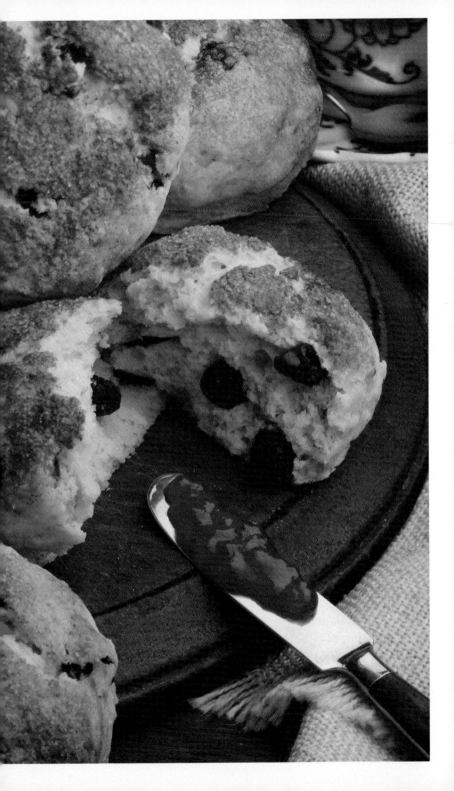

Country Scones
An English favorite for nutrition-conscious Americans!

Photo Credits
Photography by Barney Taxel
Barney Taxel & Co.
216/431-2400

Recipe Credits
Country Scones, see page 161
Servings: 24 scone wedges

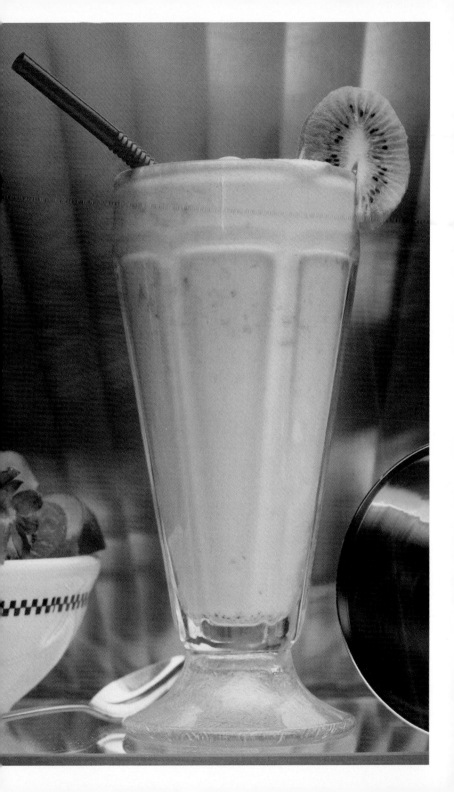

Strawberry Shake

Smooth and frothy, cool and creamy. This shake is refreshing anytime!

Photo Credits
Photography by Barney Taxel
Barney Taxel & Co.
216/431-2400

Recipe Credits
Strawberry Shake, see page 165
Servings: 4

Caribbean Pudding

SERVES 6
1 envelope unflavored gelatin
1-3/4 cups papaya nectar
2 tablespoons sugar
2 teaspoons grated lime rind
1 (8-ounce) carton plain nonfat yogurt
1 (8-ounce) can crushed pineapple in juice, drained
1/4 teaspoon coconut extract
1 medium mango (about 3/4 pound)
1 tablespoon fresh lime juice

1. Place papaya nectar in a saucepan; sprinkle gelatin over nectar and let stand 1 minute.
2. Turn heat to medium, add sugar and cook, stirring constantly until sugar and gelatin dissolve.
3. Remove mixture from heat and add lime rind.
4. Chill papaya mixture until its a syrupy consistency.
5. Add yogurt, pineapple and coconut extract; stir well.
6. Divide fruit mixture evenly among 6 dessert cups.
7. Peel and slice mango.
8. Brush with lime juice.
9. Arrange slices over each serving.

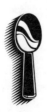

☑ Nutrition Information

Calories	122
Carbohydrates (grams)	27.9
Proteins (grams)	3.6
Cholesterol (milligrams)	1
Sodium (milligrams)	35
Fat (grams)	0.4
Saturated Fat (grams)	0

Springtime Layer Cake

SERVES 16
1 (10-3/4 ounce) loaf commercial angel food cake
1/4 cup low-sugar orange marmalade spread
1 tablespoon plus 1 teaspoon amaretto
1/4 cup low-sugar raspberry spread
1 tablespoon and 1 teaspoon amaretto
2 ounces semi-sweet chocolate

1. Scrape brown edges off cake.
2. Slice, horizontally, into 5 layers.
3. In a small bowl combine orange marmalade with 1 T plus 1 t amaretto; stir and set aside.
4. Combine same amount of amaretto with raspberry spread; stir and set aside.
5. Spread 1/2 of orange marmalade mixture on 1 cake layer; top with another cake layer.
6. Repeat procedure using raspberry mixture.
7. Repeat procedure alternating orange mixture then raspberry mixture.
8. Place layer cake in pan; cover tightly with plastic wrap and chill 10 hours. Remove cakes from pan and cut into 16 pieces.
9. Place chocolate in a ziplock freezer bag.
10. To melt chocolate, place bag in hot water. Cut a small corner off bag and drizzle chocolate over each cake.

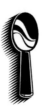

☑ Nutrition Information

Calories	75
Carbohydrates (grams)	14.4
Proteins (grams)	1.3
Cholesterol (milligrams)	0
Sodium (milligrams)	29
Fat (grams)	1.2
Saturated Fat (grams)	0.7

Almond Biscotti

YIELDS 4 DOZEN COOKIES
1/2 cup sugar
1/4 cup margarine, softened
1/2 cup egg substitute
1 teaspoon almond extract
1/4 teaspoon anise extract
1-3/4 cups all-purpose flour, divided
1/2 cup ground almonds
1 teaspoon baking powder
Vegetable cooking spray

1. Blend first 5 ingredients in a bowl.
2. Combine 1-1/2 cups flour, almonds, and baking powder.
3. Add to egg mixture and beat well with an electric mixer.
4. Stir in remaining flour; cover and chill 3 hours.
5. Coat 2 baking sheets with cooking spray.
6. Divide dough in half.
7. Place 1 half on each baking sheet.
8. Shape each half into a 10-12 inch log, about 3/4 inch thick.
9. Bake at 350 for 20 minutes; cool.
10. Slice logs into 1/4 inch slices. Place on baking sheets, cut side down and bake at 300 for 15 minutes.
11. Turn biscottis over and bake 15 minutes more.

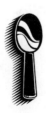

☑ *Nutrition Information*

Calories	40
Carbohydrates (grams)	6.1
Proteins (grams)	1.0
Cholesterol (milligrams)	0
Sodium (milligrams)	21
Fat (grams)	1.3
Saturated Fat (grams)	0.2

Oat Bran and Apple Waffles with Apricots

YIELDS 12 WAFFLES
1/4 cup diet margarine, softened
2 egg whites
1-1/4 cup all purpose flour
1 cup whole wheat flour
2 teaspoon baking powder
1/2 teaspoon baking soda
1/4 teaspoon salt
2 tablespoon brown sugar
1/2 teaspoon ground cinnamon
1 cup grated apple
1-3/4 cup boiling water
Nonstick cooking spray
Apricot halves, canned (about 24 halves)

1. Beat margarine with an electric mixer until fluffy. Add egg and egg whites one at a time, beating after each addition.
2. Combine all-purpose flour and next 6 ingredients, stirring well.
3. Add flour mixture to creamed mixture in the following fashion: add 1/3 of flour to creamed mixture, beat until blended; add 1/2 of water, beat until blended; add 1/3 of flour mixture, beat until blended; add 1/2 of water; beat until blended; add last 1/3 of flour mixture, beat until blended. Fold in apples.
4. Coat an 8-inch waffle iron with cooking spray. Let iron preheat.
5. Pour about 1-1/4 cups batter onto hot waffle iron; spread batter to edges.
6. Bake 7 minutes or until steaming stops.
7. Repeat with remaining batter and top with apricots.

☑ Nutrition Information

Calories	274
Carbohydrates (grams)	52
Proteins (grams)	6.8
Cholesterol (milligrams)	0
Sodium (milligrams)	354
Fat (grams)	4.5
Saturated Fat (grams)	0.8

Country Scones

YIELDS 24 SCONE WEDGES
1/2 cup dried currants or raisins
2 cups all-purpose flour • 3 tablespoons brown sugar
2 teaspoons baking powder
1/2 teaspoon baking soda • 1/3 cup diet margarine
1 8-ounce carton nonfat sour cream • 1 beaten egg yolk
1 slightly beaten egg white • 1 tablespoon water
1 tablespoon brown sugar
1/8 teaspoon ground cinnamon

1. Place currants in a small bowl; pour hot water over currants to cover; let stand 5 minutes. Drain currants and set aside.
2. In a large bowl, mix together flour, 3 tablespoons brown sugar, baking powder and baking soda. Cut in margarine.
3. Add currants and toss until mixed.
4. Make a well in the center of the dry mixture.
5. In a bowl stir together Non fat sour cream and egg yolk; add this to dry mixture and stir until moistened.
6. Lightly flour a clean cutting board. Transfer dough to cutting board and quickly knead dough by gently folding and pressing 10-12 strokes (dough should be nearly smooth).
7. Divide dough into 6 portions; shape each portion into a ball; pat each to 4 inches round and about 1/2 inch thick.
8. Place scones on a ungreased cookie sheet about 1 inch apart.
9. Cut scones into 4 wedges but do not separate wedges.
10. Brush tops of scones with mixture of egg white and water.
11. Combine 1 tablespoon brown sugar and cinnamon; sprinkle over tops of scones.
12. Bake scones in a 425 oven for 15 minutes; cool; break into wedges and serve.

☑ Nutrition Information

Calories	115
Carbohydrates (grams)	21
Proteins (grams)	2.9
Cholesterol (milligrams)	14
Sodium (milligrams)	99
Fat (grams)	1.9
Saturated Fat (grams)	0.3

Islands Afloat in a Fruity Sauce

SERVES 8

1 (16-oz) pkg. frozen unsweetened raspberries, thawed
4 cups peeled and sliced nectarines (about 1-1/2 pounds)
3 tablespoons fresh lime juice
1 tablespoon corn syrup
1 tablespoon kirsch or other cherry-flavored brandy
2 egg whites
1/4 teaspoon cream of tartar
1/4 teaspoon almond extract
1/2 cup sugar

1. In a blender process raspberries, nectarines and lime juice until smooth. Stir in corn syrup and kirsch; cover and chill.
2. Beat egg whites (which should be at room temperature) cream of tartar and almond extract until foamy.
3. Slowly add sugar, 1 tablespoon at a time; beat until stiff peaks form.
4. Pour boiling water into a baking pan to 1 inch depth.
5. Drop egg white mixture in 8 equal portions into boiling water.
6. Bake at 350 for 15 minutes or until lightly browned.
7. Remove egg white "islands" and drain; chill. Spoon raspberry mixture into 8 dessert dishes; top with an "island" and serve.

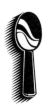

☑ Nutrition Information

Calories	142
Carbohydrates (grams)	34.2
Proteins (grams)	1.8
Cholesterol (milligrams)	0
Sodium (milligrams)	21
Fat (grams)	0
Saturated Fat (grams)	0

Peachy Kugel

SERVES 12

1 cup 1% low-fat cottage cheese
4 (8-ounce) cartons egg substitute
1 (8-ounce) carton low-fat sour cream
3/4 cup raisins
1/2 cup sugar
2 tablespoons reduced-calorie stick margarine, melted
1 teaspoon ground cinnamon
1/4 teaspoon salt
1 (16-ounce) can unsweetened sliced peaches, drained
and coarsely   chopped
8 cups cooked egg noodles (about 12 ounces uncooked)
Vegetable cooking spray
1/3 cup coarsely crushed cornflakes

1. *Combine first 9 ingredients in a bowl; stir well.*
2. *Add noodles and toss to coat.*
3. *Coat a baking dish with nonstick spray.*
4. *Transfer noodle mixture into baking dish.*
5. *Sprinkle with cornflakes.*
6. *Cover and bake in preheated 350 oven for 30 minutes.*
7. *Uncover and bake an additional 10 minutes.*

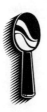

✓ Nutrition Information

Calories	270
Carbohydrates (grams)	42.9
Proteins (grams)	13.3
Cholesterol (milligrams)	8
Sodium (milligrams)	312
Fat (grams)	4
Saturated Fat (grams)	1.8

Raspberry Creme Custard Cups

SERVES 8
1/3 cup firmly packed light brown sugar
2 tablespoons cornstarch
3 egg whites, lightly beaten
1 egg, lightly beaten
1 (12-ounce) can evaporated skimmed milk
1 teaspoon vanilla extract
1 (8-ounce) tub reduced-fat cream cheese
1-1/2 cups raspberries
8 teaspoons light brown sugar

1. *Combine first 5 ingredient.*
2. *Place in the top of a double boiler.*
3. *Cook 4 minutes over simmering water, stirring constantly until thickened.*
4. *Remove from heat; add vanilla and cream cheese.*
5. *Stir until smooth; fold in raspberries.*
6. *Divide mixture evenly among 8 custard cups; cover and chill 5 hours.*
7. *Sprinkle each serving with 1 teaspoon brown sugar.*
8. *Broil 1 minute or until sugar melts; serve immediately.*

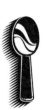

☑ Nutrition Information

Calories	177
Carbohydrates (grams)	23.4
Proteins (grams)	8.4
Cholesterol (milligrams)	46
Sodium (milligrams)	242
Fat (grams)	5.6
Saturated Fat (grams)	3.1

Strawberry Shake

SERVES 4
2 cups fresh strawberries
3 cups skim milk
1/2 cup sugar
1/4 cup egg substitute
1/4 cup instant non-fat dry milk powder
1 (12-ounce) can evaporated skimmed milk
1/2 teaspoon vanilla extract

1. *Process strawberries in a blender until smooth; chill puree at least 1 hour.*
2. *Combine milk, sugar, egg and milk powder in a saucepan; cook over medium heat, stirring constantly, until thickened.*
3. *Remove from heat and chill.*
4. *Combine strawberry puree, milk mixture, evaporated milk and vanilla in a blender.*
5. *Process until thoroughly blended.*
6. *Divide among 4 glasses.*

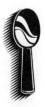

☑ Nutrition Information

Calories	79
Carbohydrates (grams)	14.4
Proteins (grams)	4.4
Cholesterol (milligrams)	1.9
Sodium (milligrams)	65
Fat (grams)	0.4
Saturated Fat (grams)	0.1

Mandarin Orange Parfaits

SERVES 4
2 cups orange sherbet
1/4 cup low-sugar orange marmalade
1 (8-ounce) carton vanilla nonfat yogurt
2 teaspoons grated orange rind

1. *Scoop 1/2 cup sherbet into each of 4 parfait glasses.*
2. *Top each with 1 tablespoon marmalade.*
3. *Spoon yogurt evenly over each.*
4. *Sprinkle 1/2 teaspoon orange rind over each parfait.*
5. *Serve immediately.*

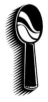

☑ **Nutrition Information**

Calories	164
Carbohydrates (grams)	38.3
Proteins (grams)	4
Cholesterol (milligrams)	10
Sodium (milligrams)	85
Fat (grams)	0
Saturated Fat (grams)	0

5
A Month of Menus

Here are 30 well-balanced meals, all of them low in saturated fat, cholesterol, sodium, and calories. Special foods are included to help reduce your cholesterol levels and body weight.

DAY ONE

Breakfast
1/2 cup orange juice
1 cup oatmeal, with 1 tablespoon raisins, and
    1/2 cup skim or low-fat milk
herbal tea or coffee

Lunch
3-4 oz canned salmon on a bed of lettuce, with
    sliced cucumbers and tomato
    1/4-1/2 cup non-fat yogurt or cottage cheese
3/4 whole rye crackers
fresh peach
iced tea or club soda

Dinner
1 cup whole wheat spaghetti, with 1/2 cup tomato sauce
    (made with olive oil) 1 teaspoon parmesan cheese
1/2 cup steamed Italian-cut beans
tossed green salad with non-fat Italian dressing
4oz dry red wine or club soda with lime

Snack
1 cup skim
1-2 graham crackers

Day Two

Breakfast
1/2 medium grapefruit
1/2 small oat bran muffin
1 cup skim milk
herbal tea or coffee

Lunch
spinach salad:
    fresh spinach leaves, with mfresh mushroom slices
    grated hard-cooked egg white
    2 anchovies topped with, olive oil-vinegar-lemon dressing
1 small whole-wheat pita pocket
1 medium apple
iced tea or club soda

Dinner
chicken stir-fry:
    1/2 cup mixed vegetables (celery, bell peppers, carrots,
    zucchini, water chestnuts, peapods, mushrooms)
    3oz chicken, cut in thin strips and stir-fried in 1-2 teaspoon
canola oil
1 cup brown rice
1/2 cup pineapple chunks
iced tea or club soda

Snack
1 cup non-fat yogurt (vanilla, coffee, or lemon-flavored)

DAY THREE

Breakfast
1/2 cup apple juice
1 cup bran cereal,
    with 1/2 banana, sliced, and 1/2 cup skim milk
herbal tea or coffee

Lunch
non-fat cream cheese and jelly sandwich:
    2 slices whole wheat bread, with
    4-5 tablespoons non-fat cream cheese
    1-4 tablespoons all-fruit strawberry preserve
1 cup skim milk
1 small box (1-1/2oz) raisins

Dinner
oysters on half shell (1 cup or 10-15) with fresh horseradish
tossed salad with low-fat dressing
1/2 steamed green beans, with
    1 teaspoon slivered almonds
1 small slice angelfood cake, with
    1/4 cup fresh strawberries
iced tea or club soda

Snack
1/4 cup hummus with vegetable sticks (celery, carrots, bell
    peppers, etc.)

Day Four

Breakfast

1/2 cup pineapple juice
1 cup hot oat bran cereal, with
   1 tablespoon raisins, and
   1/2 cup skim milk
herbal tea or coffee

Lunch

tuna fish sandwich:
   3-1/2oz canned tuna in water mixed, with
   1-2 tablespoon low-fat yogurt
   chopped celery
   green pepper
   onion, garnished, with
   lettuce leaves, on
   2 slices pumpernickel bread
1 cup skim milk
1 medium pear

Dinner

1/2 large sweet potato, baked and mashed
1/2 cup wild rice
1 cup steamed broccoli with lemon
1/4 cup fresh fruit sorbet
iced tea or club soda

Snack

2-3 cups hot-air popped popcorn, dry

DAY FIVE

Breakfast

1/2 small melon, filled with
    1/2 cup non-fat cottage cheese, and
    10-12 seedless grapes
1 slice oatmeal bread, toasted, with
    1 teaspoon marmalade or all-fruit preserve
herbal tea or coffee

Lunch

1 cup meatless chili, with
    1 teaspoon grated Parmesan cheese
3-4 whole wheat crackers
1 medium fresh tangerine
iced tea or club soda

Dinner

3-4oz broiled swordfish with lemon
1 medium red potato, baked
1 cup steamed brussel sprouts
tossed salad, with non-fat French dressing
1 cup skim milk

Snack

1 cup non-fat yogurt, with 1/2 cup blueberries

Day Six

Breakfast
1/2 cup orange juice
1 cup oat bran flakes, with
   1/2 small banana, sliced
   1/2 cup skim milk
herbal tea or coffee

Lunch
health salad:
   Romaine lettuce with sliced cucumber, red pepper, mushrooms, and
   1/2 cup bean sprouts, garnish with,
   chickpeas, kidney beans, and
   3 tablespoons slivered almonds topped, with
   olive oil-vinegar-lemon dressing
1-2 whole wheat breadsticks
2 pineapple rings
iced tea or club soda

Dinner
3oz roasted turkey breast
1/2 cup barley stuffing (made without egg yolk or butter)
1 cup steamed baby carrots with fresh mint garnish
1/2 cup baby sweet peas
baked apple with honey and raisins
iced tea or club soda

Snack
1 cup skim milk
1-2 non-fat fig cookies

Breakfast
1/2 medium grapefruit
1 egg, poached, on
    1 slice oatmeal toast
1 cup skim milk
herbal tea or coffee

Lunch
bagel broiler:
    1 whole wheat or rye bagel, broiled with
    1-1/2oz non-fat cheese and sliced tomato
1 cup fruit salad
iced tea or club soda

Dinner
baked vegetable casserole:
    1 cup chopped spinach and/or broccoli mixed, with
    1/2 cup cooked red kidney beans
    1/2 cooked brown rice, and
    sauteed onions
    garlic
    mushrooms; top with
1oz part-skim mozzarella cheese, in strips
tossed salad with low-fat dressing
1 medium nectarine
iced tea or club soda

Snack
1 light beer or 3oz dry white wine

Breakfast
1/2 cup orange juice
1 cup oatmeal, with
    1 tablespoon chopped dates, and
    1/2 cup skim milk
herbal tea or coffee

Lunch
salad nicoise:
    Romaine lettuce tossed, with
    3-1/2oz canned tuna in water
    1/2 cup white beans, wedges of tomato, and
    1 small boiled potato, cut in wedges, topped with
    non-fat Italian dressing
3-4 whole rye crackers
1 medium fresh peach
iced tea or club soda

Dinner
1 cup whole grain pasta, with
    1/2 cup tomato sauce (made with olive oil), and
    1 teaspoon grated Parmesan cheese
    1 small whole wheat roll
    1 cup steamed cauliflower with lemon
    1 cup skim milk

Snack
1 cup non-fat yogurt with
1/2 cup blueberries

Day Nine

Breakfast
1/2 medium grapefruit
1-2 small oat bran muffins
1 cup skim milk
herbal tea or coffee

Lunch
Greek salad:
    iceberg lettuce, with
    sliced mushrooms, cucumbers, tomato, and
    1oz crumbled feta cheese, and
    5 large olives, topped with
    olive oil-vinegar-lemon dressing
1 small whole wheat pita pocket
1 medium apple
iced tea or club soda

Dinner
tofu stir-fry:
    4oz tofu, sliced thin, stir-fried in
    1-2 tsp olive oil; add
    1-2 cups mixed vegetables (celery, carrots, red cabbage,
        bamboo shoots, Chinese mushrooms, green beans, and
        bok choy), on bed of
    1 cup brown rice
1/2 cup pineapple tidbits
tea or club soda

Snack
1/2 cup non-fat ice cream

DAY TEN

Breakfast

1/2 cup apple juice
1 cup bran cereal, with
    1/4 cup sliced strawberries, and
    1/2 cup skim milk
herbal tea or coffee

Lunch

non-fat cream cheese and date sandwich:
    2 slices oatmeal bread, with
    4-6 teaspoon non-fat cream cheese
    1-2 small banana, sliced thin, and
    2 dates sliced
1 cup skim milk
1 small box (1-1/2oz) raisin

Dinner

3oz roasted chicken breast without skin
tossed salad, with
    non-fat dressing
1 medium ear corn-on-the-cob
1 small slice sponge cake, with
    1/4 cup raspberries, and
1-2 tablespoons vanilla-flavored non-fat yogurt
iced tea or club soda

Snack

2-3 cups hot air popped popcorn, with
    1 teaspoon grated Parmesan cheese

DAY ELEVEN

Breakfast

1/2 cup pineapple juice
1 cup hot oat bran cereal, with
    1 tablespoon chopped dates, and
    1/2 cup skim milk
herbal tea or coffee

Lunch

seafood salad sandwich:
    3-1/2oz canned salmon (or mackerel) mixed, with
    1-2 tablespoons non-fat yogurt
    chopped onion
    celery
    carrot, and
    lettuce leaves on
    2 slices rye bread
1 cup skim milk
1 medium pear

Dinner

3oz roasted lean lamb, with
    1/2 tsp mint jelly
1/2 large sweet potato, baked and mashed
1/2 cup wild rice
1 cup steamed broccoli with pearl onions
1/2 cup fruit cocktail
iced tea or club soda

Snack

choco-shake:
    1 cup skim milk, blend with
    1 teaspoon cocoa and crushed ice, until smooth

Day Twelve

Breakfast

1 cup non-fat yogurt mixed, with
  1/2 cup fresh berries (strawberries, raspberries, and/or
      blueberries) and
  1/2 small sliced banana, and
  1 teaspoon wheat germ
1 slice toasted oatmeal bread, with
  1 teaspoon all-fruit preserve
herbal tea or coffee

Lunch

hummus sandwich:
  1/2 cup hummus in
  1 small whole wheat pita pocket, with
  cucumber, tomato slices, and lettuce
1 cup skim milk
1 medium fresh tangerine

Dinner

3-4oz broiled haddock with lemon
1 medium baked potato, with
  1 tablespoon non-fat yogurt
1 cup lima beans
1/2 cup boiled beets
1 light beer or club soda

Snack

3-4 whole grain crackers
1-1/2oz non-fat cheese
1/2 cup cider

Day Thirteen

Breakfast
1/2 cup orange juice
1 cup oat bran flakes, with
    1 sliced fresh peach, and
    1/2 cup skim milk
herbal tea or coffee

Lunch
chef's salad:
    Bibb lettuce, with
    1-2oz lean chicken or turkey strips, topped with
    non-fat Ranch-style dressing
1 small whole wheat roll
1/2 cup pineapple chunks
iced tea or club soda

Dinner
1 Boca Burger (R)
1 whole wheat bun, with
    sliced onion, tomato, and lettuce
1 cup mixed vegetables (corn, peas, carrots), steamed
1 cup skim milk
1/2 cup applesauce

Snack
1/2 cup non-fat ice cream
1oz peanuts or pecans, chopped

Day Fourteen

Breakfast

1/2 medium grapefruit
2 small buckwheat pancakes, with
    1-2 teaspoon pure maple syrup
1 cup skim milk
herbal tea or coffee

Lunch

muffin broiler:
    1 whole wheat English muffin, split;
    broil with 1-1/2 oz part-skim mozzarella cheese, topped
        with 1/4 teaspoon Dijon-style mustard
1 cup fruit salad
iced tea or club soda

Dinner

chicken with herbs:
    3 oz baked skinless chicken, with
    sliced tomato, fresh basil, tarragon
tabouleh salad:
    1 cup cracked wheat, with
    chopped tomato, fresh mint, and scant amount of olive oil
1 cup steamed zucchini with lemon
baked banana with honey
iced tea or club soda

Snack

1/4 cup hummus with vegetable sticks (celery, carrots, bell peppers, etc.)

DAY FIFTEEN

Breakfast
1/2 cup orange juice
1 cup oatmeal, with
   1 tablespoon raisins, and
   1/2 cup skim milk
herbal tea or coffee

Lunch
lobster salad:
   3-1/2oz chilled cooked lobster, on bed of lettuce, with
   sliced cucumbers and tomato, and
   1-2 tablespoons non-fat yogurt (as dressing)
3-4 whole grain sesame crackers
1 medium fresh peach
iced tea or club soda

Dinner
baked macaroni:
   1 cup whole wheat macaroni, cooked, and mixed with
   1-1/2oz non-fat cheese
   2 tsp grated Parmesan cheese
   season to taste
1 cup steamed broccoli with lemon
tossed salad with non-fat Italian dressing
1-2 fresh apricots
iced tea or club soda

Snack
1 cup non-fat yogurt, with
   1/4 cup crushed pineapple

Breakfast

1/2 medium grapefruit
1-2 small oat bran muffins
1 cup skim milk
herbal tea or coffee

Lunch

spinach salad:
    fresh spinach leaves, with
    fresh mushroom slices,
    grated hard-cooked egg whites,
    1-2 sardines, and
    non-fat Italian dressing
1-2 whole wheat breadsticks
1 medium apple
iced tea or club soda

Dinner

turkey stir-fry:
    3oz turkey, cut in strips, stir-fried in 1-2 teaspoons
        canola oil, with
    1-2 cups mixed vegetables (celery, red cabbage, zucchini,
        water chestnuts, peapods, mushrooms)
1 cup brown rice
1/2 cup fresh papaya
tea

Snack

1 cup skim milk
1-2 fig cookies

Day Seventeen

Breakfast
1/2 cup apple juice
1 cup bran cereal, with
    1/2 small banana, sliced, and
    1/2 cup skim milk
herbal tea or coffee

Lunch
non-fat ham with non-fat cheese sandwich:
    2 slices rye bread with mustard
1 cup skim milk
1 small box (1-1/2oz) raisins

Dinner
jumbo shrimp cocktail:
    1/2 cup shrimp (5-6 large), with
    1 tablespoon fresh salsa
tossed salad with non-fat dressing
1/2 cup steamed green beans, with
    1 teaspoon slivered almonds
1 small slice angelfood cake, with
    1/4 cup blueberries
iced tea or club soda

Snack
3-4 whole grain crackers, with
    1oz non-fat cheese

Day Eighteen

Breakfast

1/2 cup pineapple juice
1 cup hot oat bran cereal, with
    1 tablespoon raisins, and
    1/2 cup skim milk
herbal tea or coffee

Lunch

broiled tuna melt sandwich:
    3-1/2oz canned tuna in water, mixed with
    1-2 tablespoons non-fat yogurt
    onion powder
    garlic powder
    fresh parsley, on
    2 slices oatmeal toast, topped with
    1-1/2oz part-skim mozzarella cheese
1 medium pear
iced tea or club soda

Dinner

3oz salmon broiled
1/2 large sweet potato, baked and mashed
1/2 cup winter squash, baked and mashed
1 cup steamed cauliflower with lemon
1 small whole wheat roll
4oz dry white wine or club soda with lime

Snack

yogurt shake:
    1 cup plain non-fat yogurt, blended with
    1/2 cup fresh fruit (berries, banana, and/or peach) and
        crushed ice, until smooth

Day Nineteen

Breakfast

1/4 medium cantaloupe, filled with
    1/2 cup low-fat cottage cheese
    10-12 fresh cherries, pitted and sliced
1 slice toasted oatmeal bread, with
    1 teaspoon marmalade or all-fruit preserve
herbal tea or coffee

Lunch

1 cup meatless chili, with 1 teaspoon grated Parmesan cheese
3-4 whole wheat crackers
fresh tangerine
iced tea or club soda

Dinner

3-4oz broiled cod, with
    sliced tomato, fresh parsley
1 medium red potato, baked
1 cup corn niblets
tossed salad, with non-fat Thousand Island dressing
1 cup skim milk

Snack

1 cup non-fat yogurt (vanilla, coffee or lemon flavored)
1-2 graham crackers

Breakfast

1/2 cup orange juice
1 cup oat bran flakes, with
    1/2 small banana, sliced, and
    1/2 cup skim milk
herbal tea or coffee

Lunch

3 bean salad:
    Romaine lettuce bed, with
    1/2 cup chickpeas, kidney beans, white beans, and
    1/2 cup non-fat cottage cheese, with
        olive-vinegar-lemon dressing
1-2 whole wheat bread sticks
1/2 cup fresh mango
iced tea or club soda

Dinner

3oz baked chicken
1 medium potato, baked and mashed
1 cup steamed carrots
1/2 cup sweet peas with pearl onions
baked apple with honey and raisins
iced tea or club soda

Snack

1 cup skim milk
1 small bran muffin

Day Twenty-One

Breakfast
1/2 medium grapefruit
1 egg, poached, on 1 slice oatmeal toast
1 cup skim milk
herbal tea

Lunch
broiled pocket pizza:
    1 small whole wheat pita stuffed, with
    1-1/2oz part-skim mozzarella cheese, and
    1 medium sliced tomato
1 cup fruit salad
iced tea or club soda

Dinner
black beans and rice:
    1 cup cooked black beans, with
    1 cup cooked brown rice, sauteed onion, garlic, mushrooms
tossed salad with non-fat dressing
1 medium nectarine
iced tea or club soda

Snack
vegetable crunchies (raw carrot, celery, zucchini sticks)
1/2 cup non-fat yogurt with lemon and chives (as dip)

Breakfast
1/2 cup orange juice
1 cup oatmeal, with
    1 tablespoon chopped dates, and
    1/2 skim milk
herbal tea or coffee

Lunch
crab salad:
    1/2 cup chilled cooked crab, (fresh or canned) on bed of
        lettuce, with sliced cucumbers, cherry tomatoes, and
        dressed with 1-2 tablespoons non-fat yogurt
3-4 whole grain sesame crackers
1 medium fresh peach
iced tea or club soda

Dinner
1 cup cooked whole wheat lasagna, baked, with
    1-1/2oz non-fat cheese
    1/2 cup low-fat ricotta cheese
    1/2 cup spinach
    1/2 cup tomato sauce (made with olive oil)
tossed green salad with non-fat Italian dressing
4oz dry red wine or club soda with lemon

Snack
1/2 cup non-fat ice cream
1/4 cup berries (strawberries, raspberries, and/or blueberries)

DAY TWENTY-THREE

Breakfast
1/2 medium grapefruit
1-2 small oat bran muffins
1 cup skim milk
herbal tea or coffee

Lunch
salad nicoise:
    Romaine lettuce tossed, with
    3-1/2oz canned tuna in water
    1 medium tomato cut in wedges
    1/2 cup white beans
    1 small boiled potato, cut in wedges, topped with
    non-fat Italian dressing
1-2 whole grain breadsticks
1 medium apple
iced tea or club soda

Dinner
tofu stir-fry:
    4oz tofu, sliced thin, stir-fried in
    1-2 teaspoon olive oil, add
    1-2 cups mixed vegetables (carrots, bamboo shoots,
        Chinese mushrooms, green beans and bok choy)
1 cup brown rice
1/2 cup pineapple tidbits
tea

Snack
1 cup skim milk
1-2 oatmeal-raisin cookies

Day Twenty-Four

Breakfast
1/2 cup apple juice
1 cup bran cereal, with 1/4 cup sliced strawberries, and
   1/2 cup skim milk
herbal tea or coffee

Lunch
non-fat cream cheese and raisin sandwich:
   2 slices oatmeal bread, with 4-6 teaspoons
   non-fat cream cheese, 1 tablespoon raisins
1 cup skim milk
1 small banana

Dinner
3-4oz scallops with lemon
1/2 cup acorn squash, baked and mashed
1/2 cup steamed wax beans
tossed salad with non-fat French dressing
1/2 pear, poached in red wine
iced tea or club soda

Snack
2-3 cups hot air popped popcorn, with
   1 teaspoon grated Parmesan cheese

Day Twenty-Five

Breakfast

1-2 pineapple juice
1 cup hot oat bran cereal, with 1 tablespoon chopped dates,
    and1/2 cup skim milk
herbal tea or coffee

Lunch

salmon salad sandwich:
    3-1/2oz canned salmon, mixed with
    1-2 tablespoons non-fat yogurt, chopped onion, celery red
    bell peppers, and lettuce, on 2 slices cracked wheat bread
1 cup skim milk
1 medium pair

Dinner

1 Boca Burger®, broiled
1 medium baked potato
1/2 cup steamed brussel sprouts
1/2 cup corn niblets
1 small whole wheat roll
1 cup fresh fruit salad
iced tea or club soda

Snack

1/2 cup non-fat ice cream, with
    1/2 cup fresh strawberries

DAY TWENTY-SIX

Breakfast

1 cup non-fat yogurt, mixed with
 1/2 cup fresh berries (strawberries, raspberries, and/or
  blueberries)
 1/2 small sliced banana
 1 teaspoon wheat germ
1 slice oatmeal bread toasted, with
 1 teaspoon all-fruit preserve
herbal tea or coffee

Lunch

tomato and cheese sandwich:
 1 small whole wheat pita pocket, stuffed with
 sliced tomato
 1-1/2oz part-skim mozzarella cheese
 sprouts, topped with
 1 teaspoon non-fat mayonnaise
1 medium fresh tangerine
iced tea or club soda

Dinner

3-4oz broiled flounder or lake trout
1 medium baked red potato
1 cup steamed broccoli with lemon
tossed salad with non-fat dressing
3oz dry white wine or club soda

Snack

1 cup skim milk
1-2 oatmeal-raisin cookies

DAY TWENTY-SEVEN

Breakfast
1/2 cup orange juice
1 cup oat bran flakes, with
    1 fresh peach, sliced
    1/2 cup skim milk
herbal tea or coffee

Lunch
Antipasto salad:
    iceberg lettuce bed, with
    1-1/2oz part-skim mozzarella cheese strips
    1oz non-fat ham strips
    sliced cucumber
    tomato wedges
    5 large Greek olives
    2 anchovies, topped with
    non-fat Italian dressing
1-2 whole grain breadsticks
fresh plum
iced tea or club soda

Dinner
3oz baked chicken
1/2 cup barley stuffing (made without egg yolk or butter)
1 cup steamed baby carrots with fresh mint garnish
1/2 cup baby sweet peas
baked apple with honey and raisins
iced tea or club soda

Snack
2 rice cakes, with
    2 oz non-fat cheese

DAY TWENTY-EIGHT

Breakfast

1/2 medium grapefruit
1 medium whole wheat waffle, with
    1-2 teaspoon pure maple syrup
1 cup skim milk
herbal tea or coffee

Lunch

muffin broiler:
    1 whole wheat English muffin, split, topped with
    1-1/2oz part-skim mozzarella cheese
    thinly sliced mushrooms, onion, and green pepper
1 cup fruit salad
iced tea or club soda

Dinner

meatless chili
tossed salad with non-fat Thousand Island dressing
1 small whole wheat roll
1 medium nectarine
iced tea or club soda

Snack

1 cup non-fat yogurt (vanilla, lemon, or coffee flavored)

Day Twenty-Nine

Breakfast
1/2 cup orange juice
1-2 small oat bran muffins
1 cup skim milk
herbal tea or coffee

Lunch
2 herrings in tomato sauce
large tossed salad with non-fat Italian dressing
1/2 cup low-fat cottage cheese
1 small whole grain roll
1 cup melon balls
iced tea or club soda

Dinner
1 cup vegetarian baked beans, with 1 sliced non-fat hotdog
1 slice pumpernickel bread
1 medium ear corn-on-the-cob
1 cup steamed greens (turnip, mustard, kale) with
    fresh lemon slices
1/2 cup applesauce
iced tea or club soda

Snack
1 cup skim milk
1/2 whole wheat English muffin, with
    1 teaspoon all-fruit preserve

DAY THIRTY

Breakfast

1 cup citrus sections (orange and grapefruit)
1 egg, soft-boiled
1 slice toasted oatmeal bread
herbal tea or coffee

Lunch

1 cup low-sodium bean soup (lentil or split pea)
3-4 whole rye crackers
1 cup skim milk
1-2 fig cookies

Dinner

1-2 cups steamed mussels, in tomato sauce
   (made with olive oil)
1 thick slice Italian bread
1 cup steamed Italian-cut beans
tossed salad with non-fat dressing
1 small fresh persimmon
iced tea or club soda

Snack

1 cup skim milk
1/2 whole wheat English muffin, with
   1 teaspoon all-fruit preserve

Reprinted from *Cholesterol Cure Made Easy* by Sylvan R. Lewis, M.D., with the permission of Lifetime Books, Inc.

NUTRITIONAL COUNTER

FOOD	Serving	Cal.	Fat	S.Fat	Pro	Carb	Cho	Sod
Apple								
Fresh, with skin	1 med.	81	.5	.08	.2	21	0	0
Juice, unswt.	1 cup	116	.2	.04	.4	29	0	8
Applesauce, unswt.	1 cup	104	.2	.02	.4	27.6	0	4
Apricot								
Fresh	1 med.	36	.2	.02	.8	8.2	0	0
Canned, juice	1 cup	116	0	0	1.6	30	0	10
Canned, lt. syrp.	1 cup	150	.2	----	1.4	38	---	2
Dried, uncooked	2 each	34	0	0	.6	8.6	0	2
Nectar	1 cup	140	.2	.02	1	36	0	8
Artichoke								
Whole, cooked	2 each	106	.4	.08	5.2	24.8	0	158
Hearts, cooked	1 cup	74	.2	.06	3.6	17.4	0	110
Arugula	4 ozs.	28	.6	----	29	4.1	0	31
Asparagus, fresh, ckd.	1 cup	46	.6	.12	4.6	8	0	8
Avocado	1 med.	322	30.6	4.88	3.9	14.8	0	20
Bacon								
Canadian-style	2 ozs.	90	4	1.26	11.6	1	28	798
Cured, broiled	2 ozs.	326	28	9.86	17.2	.4	48	904
Turkey, cooked	2 ozs.	120	8	----	8	16	40	800
Banana, whole	1 med.	109	.5	.22	1.2	27.6	0	1
Barley, cooked	1/2 cup	97	.3	.07	1.8	22.2	0	2

Legend
Cal = Calories; Fat = Total Fat (grams); S.Fat = Saturated Fat (grams); Pro = Protein (grams); Carb = Carbohydrates (grams); Cho = Cholesterol (milligrams); Sod = Sodium (milligrams); ---- = nearly zero, less than .01

FOOD	Serving	Cal.	Fat	S.Fat	Pro	Carb	Cho	Sod
Bean sprouts, raw	1/2 cup	16	.1	.01	1.6	3.1	0	3
Beans, cooked & drained								
Black	1/3 cup	74	.3	.78	4.9	13.3	0	.7
Cannellini	1/3 cup	73	.2	.04	5	13.2	0	1.4
Garbanzo	1/3 cup	87	1.4	.14	6	14.6	0	3.9
Great Northern	1/3 cup	86	.3	.10	.8	15.4	0	1.4
Green, fresh	1/3 cup	14	.13	.03	.8	3.2	0	1.4
Green, canned	1/3 cup	9.1	0	0	.5	2	0	111
Kidney or red	1/3 cup	73	.26	.04	5	13.1	0	1.4
Lima, frzn, baby	1/3 cup	61	.19	.04	3.9	11.3	0	17.0
Pinto, canned	1/3 cup	61	.26	.05	3.6	11.3	0	120
Wax, canned	1/3 cup	9.1	0	0	.52	2	0	111
White	1/3 cup	8.3	.4	.10	5.2	15.1	0	1.3
Beef, trimmed of fat								
Flank steak, broiled	4 ozs	276	16.9	7.2	28.8	0	80	95
Ground,extra-lean,broiled	4 ozs	291	18.5	7.3	28.7	0	94.7	80
Liver, braised	4 ozs	183	5.6	2.2	27.6	3.9	441	80
Round,bottom, braised	4 ozs	252	10.9	3.9	35.9	0	109	57
Round, eye of, cooked	4 ozs	208	7.3	2.8	32.9	0	78.7	71
Round,top,lean, broil	4 ozs	216	7.1	2.5	36	0	94.7	69
Sirloin, broiled	4 ozs	236	9.9	4.04	34.4	0	101	75
Tenderloin, roasted	4 ozs	231	10.5	4.12	32	0	95	72
Beets								
Fresh, diced, cooked	1/2 cup	26	.4	.01	.9	5.7	0	42
Canned,reg. pck	1/2 cup	31	.1	.02	.8	7.5	0	201
Blueberries, fresh	1/2 cup	41	.3	.02	.5	10.2	0	4
Bouillon, dry								
Beef-flav. cubes	1 cube	3	0	----	.1	.2	---	400
Beef-flav. granls	1 tb.sp.	30	3.3	.90	1.5	1.5	---	2835

FOOD	Serving	Cal.	Fat	S.Fat	Pro	Carb	Cho	Sod
Chicken-flav. cubes	1 cube	10	.2	----	.7	1.1	--	1152
Chick-flav. granules	1 tb.sp.	30	3.3	.90	1.5	1.5	--	2457
Bran								
Oat, dry, unckd.	1/3 cup	100	2.6	.18	5.2	15.3	0	.7
Oat, unprcssd.	1/3 cup	74	2.9	.40	5.2	20	0	1.3
Wheat, crude	1/3 cup	42	.8	.12	3.1	12.6	0	.7
Bread								
Bagel, plain	2 ozs	161	1.5	.21	5.9	30.5	---	196
Biscuit,homemd.	1 each	127	6.4	1.74	2.3	14.9	2	224
Bun, hamburger /hotdog	1 each	136	3.4	.52	3.2	22.4	13	112
Cornbread	2 oz sq.	154	6	3.36	3.5	21.1	56	273
English muffin	1/2	91	1.8	.97	2.9	15.5	16	117
French	1 slice	73	.5	.16	2.3	13.9	1	145
Light	1 slice	40	1	----	2	7	0	105
Pumpernickel	1 oz	76	.4	.05	2.8	16.4	0	176
Rye	1 oz	61	.3	.04	2.3	13	0	139
White	1 oz	67	.8	.19	2.2	12.6	1	127
Whole wheat	1 oz	56	.7	.12	2.4	11	1	121
Breadcrumbs								
Fine, dry	1 cup	392	4.4	1.04	12.6	73.4	4	736
Seasoned	1 cup	428	3	----	16.8	83	---	3180
Breadstick, pln.	1 each	17	0.5	----	.4	2.7	---	20
Broccoli, fresh, chopped, cooked or raw	1/2 cup	12	.1	.02	1.3	2.3	0	12
Broth								
Beef, canned, diluted	4 ozs	16	.4	.17	2.4	1.3	12	391
Beef, no salt added	4 ozs	11	.6	.17	.3	1	0	4
Chicken, low-sodium	4 ozs	11	0	---	.2	1	0	16
Chicken,no-salt added	4 ozs	8	.5	---	.5	0	---	34

FOOD	Serving	Cal.	Fat	S.Fat	Pro	Carb	Cho	Sod
Brussel sprts. fresh cooked	1/2 cup	30	.4	.08	2	6.8	0	16
Butter								
Regular	1 tsp	34	3.8	2.4	.3	0	10.3	39
Whipped	1 tsp	27	2.6	1.6	.3	0	7	26
Cabbage								
Bok choy	1/2 cup	5	0	.01	.5	.8	0	23
Common raw, shredded	1 cup	16	.2	.02	.8	3.8	0	12
Cake, w/out frosting								
Angel food	3oz slice	220	.2	----	4.8	50.6	0	125
Pound	1oz slice	305	17.5	10.19	3.6	33.7	134	245
Sponge, cut into 8 slices	1 slice	274	7.5	2.2	5.4	46.2	332	149
Candy								
Hard	1 each	27	0	0	0	6.8	0	2
Jelly beans	1 ounce	104	.1	.09	0	26.4	0	3
Milk chocolate	1 ounce	153	8.7	5.13	2.4	16.4	7	23
Cantaloupe raw, diced	1 cup	5.6	.4	.24	1.7	13.4	0	14
Carambola (starfruit)	1 med.	42	.4	----	.7	9.9	0	3
Carrot								
Raw	1 small	25	.1	.01	.4	6.3	0	20
Cooked, sliced	1 cup	66	.2	.44	1.6	15.2	0	96
Catsup								
Regular	2 tbsp.	36	0.2	.02	0.6	8.6	0	356
Reduced-calorie	2 tbsp.	14	0	---	0	2.4	---	6
Cauliflower, raw	1 cup	24	.2	.02	2	5	0	14
Celery, raw	1 stalk	10	.1	.02	.4	2.2	0	52
Cereal								
Bran flakes	1 cup	128	.8	.12	5.0	30.6	0	364
Corn flakes	1 cup	88	0	0	1.8	19.6	0	280

FOOD	Serving	Cal.	Fat	S.Fat	Pro	Carb	Cho	Sod
Puffed rice	1 cup	44	.2	.02	1.8	9.6	0	0
Raisin Bran	1 cup	144	.1	----	5.4	3.72	0	358
Shredded mini-wheat	1 cup	152	1.0	.16	4.6	34	0	4
Cheerios	1 cup	88	1.4	.26	3.4	15.6	0	146
Whole-grain wheat flakes	1 cup	158	.4	.08	3.8	37.2	0	300

Cheese

FOOD	Serving	Cal.	Fat	S.Fat	Pro	Carb	Cho	Sod
American, processed	1 oz	106	8.9	5.58	6.3	0.5	27	405
American, processed, skim	1 oz	69	4	----	6	2	15	407
Blue	1 oz	100	8.1	5.3	6.1	.7	21	395
Brie	1 oz	95	7.8	4.94	5.9	.1	28	178
Cheddar	1 oz	114	9.4	5.98	7	.4	30	176
Cheddar, 40% less fat	1 oz	71	4.1	2.40	5	6	15	195
Cheddar, light, processed	1 oz	50	2	----	6.9	1	----	442
Cheddar, reduced-fat, sharp	1 oz	86	5.4	3.15	8.3	1.2	19	205
Colby, reduced-fat	1 oz	85	5.5	3.23	8.2	.7	19	163
Cottage, nonfat	1/4 cup	35	0	0	7.5	1.5	3	210
Cottage, low-fat, (1% milkfat)	1/4 cup	40	.6	.36	7	1.5	3	230
Cottage, low-fat, (2% milkfat)	1/4 cup	51	1.1	.70	7.8	2	5	230
Cottage (4% milkfat)	1/4 cup	54	2.4	1.5	6.6	1.4	8	213
Cream, light	2 ozs	124	9.6	5.72	5.8	3.9	32	320
Cream, nonfat	2 ozs	48	0	----	8.0	2	10	340
Feta	1 oz	75	6	4.24	4	1.2	25	316
Monterey Jack	1 oz	106	8.6	5.41	6.9	.2	22	152
Monterey Jack, reduced fat	1 oz	83	5.4	3.15	8.4	.5	19	181
Mozzarella, part-skim	1 oz	72	4.5	2.86	6.9	.8	16	132
Mozzarella, whole milk	1 oz	80	6.1	3.73	5.5	.6	22	106
Muenster	1 oz	104	8.5	5.42	6.6	.3	27	178
Neufchatel	1 oz	74	6.6	4.20	2.8	.8	22	113

FOOD	Serving	Cal.	Fat	S.Fat	Pro	Carb	Cho	Sod
Parmesan, grated	1 oz	129	8.5	5.40	11.8	1.1	22	528
Ricotta, nonfat	1 oz	20	0	----	4.0	2.0	3	15
Ricotta, part-skim	1 oz	39	2.2	1.39	3.2	1.5	9	35
Swiss	1 oz	107	7.8	5.04	8.1	1	26	74
Swiss, reduced-fat	1 oz	85	5	2.78	9.6	.5	18	44

Cherries

FOOD	Serving	Cal.	Fat	S.Fat	Pro	Carb	Cho	Sod
Fresh, sweet	1 cup	104	1.4	.32	.8	24	0	0
Sour, light syrup	1/2 cup	94	.1	.03	.9	24.3	0	9
Sour, unswtnd.	1 cup	78	.4	.10	1.6	18.8	0	4

Chicken, skinned, boned and roasted

FOOD	Serving	Cal.	Fat	S.Fat	Pro	Carb	Cho	Sod
White meat	4 ozs	196	5.1	1.43	34.7	0	96	87
Dark meat	3 ozs	174	8.3	2.26	23.3	0	79	79
Liver	3 ozs	134	4.6	1.56	20.7	.7	537	43

Chili sauce

FOOD	Serving	Cal.	Fat	S.Fat	Pro	Carb	Cho	Sod
	1 teasp.	6	0	.01	.1	1.4	0	76

Chives

FOOD	Serving	Cal.	Fat	S.Fat	Pro	Carb	Cho	Sod
raw, chopped	1 tblsp.	1	0	0	.1	.1	0	0

Chocolate

FOOD	Serving	Cal.	Fat	S.Fat	Pro	Carb	Cho	Sod
Chips, semiswt	1/4 cup	215	15.2	----	1.7	24.2	0	1
Sweet	1 oz	150	9.9	----	1.2	16.4	0	9
Unsweetened, baking	2 ozs	282	24.4	17.6	6.2	17	0	2

Chutney, apple

FOOD	Serving	Cal.	Fat	S.Fat	Pro	Carb	Cho	Sod
	1 tblspn.	41	0	----	.2	10.5	---	34

Clams

FOOD	Serving	Cal.	Fat	S.Fat	Pro	Carb	Cho	Sod
Raw	1/2 cup	92	1.2	.12	15.8	3.2	42	69
Canned, drained	1/2 cup	118	1.6	.15	20.4	4.1	54	90

Cocoa powder, unsweetened

FOOD	Serving	Cal.	Fat	S.Fat	Pro	Carb	Cho	Sod
	1 teasp.	8	.2	.15	.5	.8	0	1

Coconut

FOOD	Serving	Cal.	Fat	S.Fat	Pro	Carb	Cho	Sod
Dried, swtnd. shredded	1/2 cup	232	16.4	14.5	1.4	22	0	121
Dried, unswtnd. shredded	1/2 cup	263	25.7	22.8	2.8	9.4	0	15

FOOD	Serving	Cal.	Fat	S.Fat	Pro	Carb	Cho	Sod
Cookies								
Brownie	2 oz bar	243	10.1	3.13	2.7	39	10	153
Chocolate	3 each	216	10.2	2.7	3	28.2	39	183
Chocolate chip	3 each	156	8.7	3.3	1.8	18.6	15	87
Fig bar	3 each	180	3	.18	1.5	33	---	180
Fortune	3 each	69	.6	----	.9	15	---	---
Gingersnaps	3 each	108	3.9	.99	1.5	16.2	9	33
Oatmeal, plain	3 each	171	8.1	2	2.7	21.6	27	138
Sugar wafers	3 each	141	7.2	1.4	1.8	17.7	21	183
Vanilla wafers	3 each	51	2.7	.5	.6	6.3	6	66
Corn								
Fresh, on the cob, cooked	6 inch	89	1	.16	2.6	20.6	0	14
Cream-style, regular pack	1/2 cup	92	.5	.08	2.2	23.2	0	365
Couscous								
cooked	1 cup	200	.2	0.06	6.8	41.5	0	8
Crab								
Blue, cooked	4 ozs	116	2	.25	22.4	0	113	316
Imitation	4 ozs	116	1.5	----	13.6	11.6	23	953
King, cooked	4 ozs	109	1.7	.15	.22	0	60	1216
Crackers								
Graham, plain	2 sqrs.	60	1.0	----	1	11	---	96
Melba rounds, plain	6 each	77	1.2	----	2.4	12	---	204
Saltine	6 each	78	2.4	----	1.8	12.6	---	258
Wheat thins, reduced fat	18 each	120	4	.5	2	21	0	220
Cranberry								
Fresh, whole	1/2 cup	23	.1	.01	.2	6	0	0
Juice cocktail, reduced-calorie	1 cup	44	0	0	0	11.2	0	8
Juice cocktail, regular	1/2 cup	75	.1	0	0	19.2	0	5
Sauce, swtnd.	1/4 cup	105	.1	.01	.1	26.9	0	20
Cream								
Half-and-half	1 teasp.	7	.6	.4	.1	.2	2	2
Sour	1 tblsp.	31	3	1.88	.5	.6	6	8

FOOD	Serving	Cal.	Fat	S.Fat	Pro	Carb	Cho	Sod
Sour, nonfat	1 tblsp.	10	0	----	1	1	0	10
Whipping	1 tblsp.	51	5.5	3.43	.3	.4	20	6
Creamer,								
non-dairy, pwdr	1 teasp.	11	.7	.64	.1	1.1	0	4
Croutons,								
seasoned	1 oz	139	5	----	3	18.9	---	---
Cucumbers,								
raw, whole	1 med.	32	.3	.08	1.3	7.1	0	5
Currants	3 tblsp.	75	0	0	1.2	20.1	0	3
Dates, pitted,								
unsweetened	5 each	114	.2	.08	.8	30.5	0	1
Egg								
White	1 each	16	0	0	3.4	.3	0	52
Whole	1 each	77	5.2	1.61	6.5	.6	213	66
Yolk	1 each	61	5.2	1.62	2.8	.3	214	7
Substitute, frzn	1/4 cup	30	0	0	6	1	0	90
Eggplant,								
cooked, not salt	1 cup	26	.2	.04	0.8	6.4	0	2
Figs								
Fresh	2 med.	74	.4	.06	.8	19.8	0	2
Dried	2 each	96	.4	.08	1.2	24.4	0	4
Fish, cooked								
Flounder	4 ozs	133	1.7	.41	27.3	0	77	119
Grouper	4 ozs	133	1.5	.33	28.1	0	53	60
Haddock	4 ozs	126	1.1	.19	27.5	0	84	99
Halibut	4 ozs	159	3.3	.47	30.2	0	47	79
Mackerel,								
Spanish	4 ozs	179	7.2	2.04	26.8	0	83	75
Mahimahi	4 ozs	124	1.1	.27	26.9	0	107	128
Perch	4 ozs	133	1.3	.27	28.1	0	131	89
Pollock	4 ozs	133	1.5	.19	28	0	103	125
Pompano	4 ozs	238	13.7	5.10	27	0	72	87
Salmon, sockeye	4 ozs	245	12.4	2.17	31	0	99	75
Scamp	4 ozs	133	1.5	.33	28	0	53	60
Snapper	4 ozs	145	2	.41	30	0	53	64

FOOD	Serving	Cal.	Fat	S.Fat	Pro	Carb	Cho	Sod
Sole	4 ozs	133	1.7	.41	27	0	77	119
Swordfish	4 ozs	176	5.9	1.6	29	0	57	131
Trout, rainbow	4 ozs	171	4.9	.95	30	0	83	39
Tuna, yellowfin	4 ozs	157	1.3	.35	34	0	65	53
Tuna, canned in oil, drained	4 ozs	224	9.3	1.73	33	0	20	401
Tuna, white, in water	4 ozs	155	2.8	.75	30	0	48	444

Frankfurter

FOOD	Serving	Cal.	Fat	S.Fat	Pro	Carb	Cho	Sod
Beef	1 each	139	12.6	5.30	5.3	.7	27	451
Turkey	1 each	103	8.5	2.65	5.6	1.1	42	488

Fruit bar, frzn

FOOD	Serving	Cal.	Fat	S.Fat	Pro	Carb	Cho	Sod
	1 each	41	0	.01	.9	9.7	0	10

Fruit cocktail,

FOOD	Serving	Cal.	Fat	S.Fat	Pro	Carb	Cho	Sod
canned, in juice	1 cup	114	0	0	1.2	29.2	0	10

Gelatin
Flavored, prepared

FOOD	Serving	Cal.	Fat	S.Fat	Pro	Carb	Cho	Sod
with water	1/2 cup	81	0	----	1.5	18.6	0	54
Unflavored	1 tblsp.	30	0	----	5.2	0	---	6

Grape juice,

FOOD	Serving	Cal.	Fat	S.Fat	Pro	Carb	Cho	Sod
Concord	1/3 cup	40	0	----	0	9.7	---	7

Grapefruit

FOOD	Serving	Cal.	Fat	S.Fat	Pro	Carb	Cho	Sod
Fresh	1 med.	39	.1	.01	.8	9.7	0	0
Juice, unswtnd	1/2 cup	47	.1	.02	.6	11.1	0	1

Grapes

FOOD	Serving	Cal.	Fat	S.Fat	Pro	Carb	Cho	Sod
green,seedless	1 cup	114	.9	.30	1.1	28.4	0	3

Ham
Cured, roasted,

FOOD	Serving	Cal.	Fat	S.Fat	Pro	Carb	Cho	Sod
extra-lean	3 ozs	123	4.7	1.54	17.8	1.3	45	1023
Reduced fat, low-salt	3 ozs	104	4.2	----	15.3	1.8	42	658

Hominy

FOOD	Serving	Cal.	Fat	S.Fat	Pro	Carb	Cho	Sod
white or yellow	1/2 cup	58	.7	.10	1.2	11.4	0	168

Honey

FOOD	Serving	Cal.	Fat	S.Fat	Pro	Carb	Cho	Sod
	1 tblsp.	64	0	0	.1	17.5	0	1

FOOD	Serving	Cal.	Fat	S.Fat	Pro	Carb	Cho	Sod
Honeydew								
raw, diced	1 cup	59	.2	.08	.8	15.6	0	17
Horseradish,								
prepared	1 tblsp.	6	0	.01	.2	1.4	0	14
Hot sauce,								
bottle	1 tsp.	0	0	----	0	0	0	36
Ice cream,								
vanilla, regular	1/2 cup	134	7.2	4.39	2.3	15.9	30	58
Ice milk, vanilla	1/2 cup	92	2.8	1.76	2.6	14.5	9	52
Jams								
Regular	1 tblsp.	54	0	.01	.1	14	0	2
Reduced-calorie	1 tblsp.	29	0	----	.1	7.4	0	16
Jicama	1 cup	49	.2	.07	1.6	10.5	0	7
Kiwi	1 each	44	.5	.08	1.0	8.9	0	0
Kumquat	1 each	12	0	0	.2	3.1	0	1
Lamb								
Ground, cooked	4 ozs	321	22.3	9.2	28	0	109	92
Leg, roasted	4 ozs	216	8.8	3.1	32	0	101	77
Loin or chop,								
broiled	4 ozs	245	11.1	3.9	34	0	108	95
Rib, broiled	4 ozs	267	14.7	5.3	31	0	103	96
Lemon								
Fresh	1 each	22	.3	.04	1.3	11.4	0	3
Juice	1 tblsp.	3	0	.01	.1	1	0	3
Lentils, cooked	1/3 cup	75	.3	.03	5.8	13	0	1.3
Lettuce								
Belgian endive	1 cup	14	.1	.02	.9	2.9	0	6
Boston or Bibb,								
shredded	1 cup	7	.1	.02	0.7	1.3	0	3
Curly endive								
or escarole	1 cup	8	.1	.02	.6	1.7	0	11
Iceberg,								
chopped	1 cup	7	.1	.01	.5	1.1	0	5

FOOD	Serving	Cal.	Fat	S.Fat	Pro	Carb	Cho	Sod
Radicchio, raw	1 oz	7	.1	----	.4	1.3	0	6
Romaine, chopped	1 cup	9	.1	.01	.9	1.3	0	4

Lime

Fresh	1 each	20	.1	.01	.4	6.8	0	1
Juice	1 tblsp.	4	0	0	.1	1.4	0	0

Lobster, cooked,

meat only	4 ozs	111	0.7	0.12	23.2	1.46	81	430

Luncheon meats

Bolgna, all meat	1 oz	90	8	3.01	3.3	.8	16	289
Turkey ham	1 oz	34	1.2	.45	5.5	.3	19	286

Mango, raw

	1/2 cup	54	.2	.05	.4	14	0	2

Margarine

Regular	1 tsp	34	3.8	.74	0	0	0	44
Reduced-calorie stick	1 tsp	17	1.9	.31	0	0	0	46

Mayonnaise

Regular	1 tblsp.	99	10.9	1.62	0.2	.4	8	78
Nonfat	1 tblsp.	12	0	----	0	3	0	190
Reduced-calorie	1 tblsp.	44	4.6	.70	.1	.7	6	88

Milk

Buttermilk	1 cup	98	2.1	1.35	7.8	11.7	10	257
Buttermilk, nonfat	1 cup	88	.8	.64	8.8	12	8	256
Chocolate, low-fat 1%	1 cup	158	2.5	1.55	8.1	26.1	8	153
Condensed, sweetened	1 cup	982	26.3	16.77	24.2	166.5	104	389
Evaporated, skim canned	1 cup	200	.5	.31	19.3	29.1	10	294
Low-fat, 1% fat	1 cup	102	2.5	1.61	8	11.6	10	122
Low-fat, 2% fat	1 cup	122	4.7	2.93	8.1	11.7	20	122
Nonfat dry	1/3 cup	145	.3	.20	14.5	20.8	8	214
Skim	1 cup	86	.4	.28	8.3	11.9	5	127
Whole	1 cup	149	8.1	5.05	8	11.3	34	120

Molasses,

cane, light	1 tblsp.	52	0	----	0	13.3	0	3

FOOD	Serving	Cal.	Fat	S.Fat	Pro	Carb	Cho	Sod
Mushrooms								
Fresh	1/2 cup	9	.1	.02	0.7	1.6	0	1
Canned	1/2 cup	19	.2	.02	1.5	3.9	0	---
Mussels,								
blue, cooked	3 ozs	146	3.8	.72	20.2	6.3	43	314
Mustard								
Dijon	1 tsp	6	.3	----	0	.3	0	149
Prepared, yellow	1 tsp	4	.2	0	.2	.3	0	65
Nectarine, frsh	1 med.	67	.6	.07	1.3	16.1	0	0
Nuts								
Almonds, chpd.	1 tblsp.	48	4.2	.40	1.6	1.7	0	1
Cashews, dry, no								
salt, roasted	1 tblsp.	49	4	.78	1.3	2.8	0	1
Macadamia, no								
salt, roasted	1 tblesp.	60	6.4	.96	.6	1.1	0	1
Peanuts, roasted,								
unsalted	1 tblsp.	53	4.5	.62	2.4	1.7	0	1
Pecans, chpd.	1 tblsp.	50	5	.40	.6	1.4	0	0
Pine	1 tblsp.	52	5.1	.78	2.4	1.4	0	0
Walnuts, black	1 tblsp.	47	4.4	.28	1.9	.9	0	0
Oats								
Cooked	1/2 cup	73	1.2	.21	3.1	12.7	0	187
Rolled, dry	1 cup	312	5.2	.90	13	54.2	0	4
Oil								
Canola	1 tblsp.	117	13.6	.97	0	0	0	0
Corn	1 tblsp.	121	13.6	1.73	0	0	0	0
Olive	1 tblsp.	119	13.5	1.82	0	0	0	0
Peanut	1 tblsp.	119	13.5	2.28	0	0	0	0
Safflower	1 tblsp.	121	13.6	1.24	0	0	0	0
Sesame	1 tblsp.	121	13.6	1.92	0.0	0	0	0
Okra, cooked	1/2 cup	26	.1	.04	1.5	5.8	0	4
Olives								
Green, stuffed	1 each	4	.4	----	0	.1	---	290
Ripe	1 med.	5	.4	.08	0	.3	0	35
Onions								
Green, chopped	1 tblsp.	2	0	0	.1	.5	0	1

FOOD	Serving	Cal.	Fat	S.Fat	Pro	Carb	Cho	Sod
Raw, chopped	1/2 cup	32	.1	.02	1.0	7.3	0	3
Cooked, yellow or white	1/2 cup	23	.1	.02	.7	5.3	0	2
Orange								
Fresh	1 med.	62	.2	.02	1.2	15.4	0	0
Juice	1 cup	112	.2	.02	1.6	26.8	0	2
Mandarin, canned, packed in juice	1/2 cup	46	0	0	0.7	12.0	0	6
Mandarin, canned, packed in water	1/2 cup	37	0	----	0	8.4	----	11
Oysters, raw	3 ozs	59	2.1	.54	6	3.3	47	95
Papaya								
Fresh, cubed	1/2 cup	27	.1	.03	.4	6.9	0	2
Nectar, canned	1/2 cup	71	.3	.06	.3	18.1	0	6
Parsnips, cooked, diced	1/2 cup	63	.2	.04	1.0	15.1	0	8
Pasta, cooked								
Macaroni	1 cup	198	1	.14	6.6	39.6	0	2
Medium egg noodles	1 cup	212	2.4	.5	7.6	39.8	5.2	12
Rice noodles	1 cup	176	2.6	----	6.2	57.2	0	---
Spaghetti	1 cup	198	1.0	.14	6.6	39.6	0	2
Spinach noodles	1 cup	200	2.0	.30	7.6	37.8	0	44
Whole wheat	1 cup	200	2.8	.36	7.4	39.6	0	2
Peaches								
Fresh	1 small	37	.1	.01	.6	9.7	0	0
Canned, packed in juice	1/2 cup	55	0	0	.8	14.3	0	5
Canned, packed in light syrup	1/2 cup	69	0	0	.6	18.6	0	6
Juice	1/2 cup	57	0	----	0	13.6	---	5
Peanut butter, regular	1 tblsp.	95	8.3	1.38	4.6	2.6	0	79
Pear								
Fresh	1 med.	97	.7	.03	.6	24.9	0	0
Canned, packed in juice	1/2 cup	62	.1	0	.4	16	0	5

FOOD	Serving	Cal.	Fat	S.Fat	Pro	Carb	Cho	Sod
Canned, packed								
in light syrup	1/2 cup	71	0	----	.2	19.6	0	6
Nectar, canned	1/3 cup	48	.13	----	.3	10.5	---	1
Peas								
Black-eyed,								
cooked	1/2 cup	90	.7	.17	6.7	15	0	3
English, cooked	1/2 cup	62	.2	.04	4.1	11.4	0	70
Snow pea pods,								
cooked or raw	1/2 cup	34	.2	.03	2.6	5.6	0	3
Split, cooked	1/2 cup	116	.4	.05	8.2	20.7	0	2
Peppers								
Jalapeno, green	1 each	4	0	0	.2	.9	0	1
Sweet, raw, green,								
red or yellow	1 small	19	.4	.05	.6	3.9	0	2
Pickle								
Dill, sliced	1/4 cup	4	.1	.02	.2	.9	0	553
Sweet, sliced	1/4 cup	57	.2	.04	.2	14.1	0	276
Pie, baked,								
9-inch diameter, cut into 8 slices								
Apple, fresh	1 slice	409	15.3	5.22	3.3	67.7	12	229
Chocolate								
meringue	1 slice	354	13.4	5.38	6.8	53.8	109	307
Pecan	1 slice	478	20.3	4.31	5.8	71.1	141	324
Pumpkin	1 slice	181	6.8	2.24	4	27	61	210
Pimiento, diced	1 tblsp.	4	.1	.01	0.2	1	0	3
Pineapple								
Fresh, diced	1/2 cup	38	.3	.02	.3	9.6	0	1
Canned, packed								
in juice	1/2 cup	75	.1	.01	.5	19.6	0	1
Canned, packed								
in light syrup	1/2 cup	66	.2	.01	.5	16.9	0	1
Juice, unswtnd.	1 cup	140	.2	.02	.8	34.4	0	2
Plum, fresh	1 med.	35	.4	.03	.5	8.3	0	0
Popcorn								
hot-air popped	3 cups	70	.9	.12	2.4	13.8	0	0
Poppy seeds	1 tblsp.	47	3.9	.43	1.6	2.1	0	2

FOOD	Serving	Cal.	Fat	S.Fat	Pro	Carb	Cho	Sod
Pork, cooked								
Chop, cntr-loin	4 ozs	272	14.8	----	32.3	0	103	79
Roast	4 ozs	272	15.6	5.4	30.3	0	103	79
Tenderloin	4 ozs	188	5.5	1.9	32.7	0	105	78
Potatoes								
Baked, with skin	1 large	218	.2	.05	4.4	50.4	0	16
Boiled, diced	1/2 cup	67	.1	.02	1.3	15.6	0	4
Potato chips,								
regular	10 each	105	7.1	1.81	1.3	10.4	0	94
Pretzel sticks,								
thin	10 each	25	.5	----	.5	4.4	---	83
Prunes								
Dried, pitted	1 each	20	0	0	.2	5.3	0	0
Juice	1/2 cup	91	0	0	.8	22.3	0	5
Pumpkin, can	1/2 cup	42	.3	.18	1.3	9.9	0	6
Radish,								
fresh, sliced	1/2 cup	10	.3	0	.3	2.1	0	14
Raisins	1 tblsp.	27	0	.01	.3	7.2	0	1
Raspberries								
Black, fresh	1/2 cup	33	.4	.01	.6	7.7	0	0
Red, fresh	1/2 cup	30	.3	.01	.6	7.1	0	0
Rhubarb								
Raw, diced	1/2 cup	13	.1	.02	.5	2.8	0	2
Cooked, w/sugar	1/2 cup	157	.1	.01	.5	42.1	0	1
Rice, cooked without salt or fat								
Brown	1/3 cup		.6	----	1.6	15.1	0	0
White, lng-grain	1/3 cup	71	.1	.04	1.3	15.6	0	0
Wild	1/3 cup	54	.2	.03	2.1	11.4	0	1
Rice cake, plain	3 each	108	.6	0	2.1	23.1	0	0
Roll								
Croissant	1 each	272	17.3	10.67	4.6	24.6	47	384
Hard	1 each	156	1.6	.35	4.9	29.8	2	312
Kaiser, small	1 each	92	1.8	----	3	16	---	192

FOOD	Serving	Cal.	Fat	S.Fat	Pro	Carb	Cho	Sod
Plain	1 each	82	2.0	.34	2.2	13.7	2	141
Whole wheat	1 each	72	1.8	.51	2.3	12	9	149
Salad dressing								
Blue cheese	1 tblsp.	28	3.1	----	.1	.1	0	72
Blue cheese, low cal.	1 tblsp.	20	1.9	.5	.3	.3	4	57
Catalina, fat-free	1 tblsp.	5	0	0	0	1	0	40
French	1 tblsp.	32	3.1	----	.1	1	2	68
French, low-cal.	1 tblsp.	7	0	0	0	1.3	0	40
Italian	1 tblsp.	28	3.1	----	0	.2	0	57
Italian, no-oil, low-calorie	1 tblsp.	3	0	----	0	.6	0	54
Ranch, fat-free	1 tblsp.	5	0	0	0	1	0	50
Thousand Island	1 tblsp.	20	1.9	.31	0	.8	---	36
Thousand Island fat-free	1 tblsp.	7	0	0	0	1.7	0	45
Thousand Island, low-cal.	1 tblsp.	8	.5	.10	0	.8	1	51
Scallops, raw, large	3 ozs	75	0.6	.07	14.3	2	28	137
Sesame seeds, dry	1 tblsp.	51	4.5	.63	1.5	2.1	0	0
Sherbet								
Lime or raspberry	1/2 cup	104	0.9	----	.9	23.8	0	67
Orange	1/2 cup	135	1.9	1.19	1.1	29.3	7	44
Shrimp								
Fresh, cooked, peeled and deveined	3 ozs	84.9	.25	17	.8	0	166	191
Canned, drained	3 ozs	102	1.7	.32	19.6	.9	147	144
Soup, condensed, made with water								
Chicken noodle	1 cup	75	2.4	.65	4	9.3	7	1106
Cream of chicken	1 cup	117	7.3	2.07	2.9	9	10	986
Cream of mushroom	1 cup	129	9	2.44	2.3	9	2	1032
Cream of potato	1 cup	73	2.3	1.22	1.7	11	5	1000
Tomato	1 cup	85	1.9	.37	2	16.6	0	871
Vegetable, beef	1 cup	78	2	.83	5.4	9.8	5	956

FOOD	Serving	Cal.	Fat	S.Fat	Pro	Carb	Cho	Sod
Soy sauce								
Regular	1 tblsp.	8	0	0	.8	1.2	0	829
Low-sodium	1 tblsp.	6	0	0	0	0	0	390
Reduced-sodium	1 tblsp.	8	0	0	.8	1.2	0	484
Spinach								
Fresh	1 cup	12	.2	.03	1.6	2.0	0	44
Cooked	1/2 cup	21	.2	.04	2.7	3.4	0	63
Squash, cooked								
Acorn	1/2 cup	57	.1	.03	1.1	14.9	0	1
Butternut	1/2 cup	41	.1	.02	.8	10.7	0	4
Spaghetti	1/2 cup	22	.2	.05	.5	5	0	14
Summer	1/2 cup	18	.3	.06	.8	3.9	0	1
Strawberries,								
fresh	1 cup	45	.6	.03	.9	10.5	0	1
Sugar								
Granulated	1 tblsp.	48	0	0	0	12.4	0	0
Brown, packed	1 tblsp.	51	0	----	0	13.3	0	4
Powdered	1 tblsp.	29	0	0	0	7.5	0	0
Sweet potatoes								
Whole, baked	1/2 cup	103	.1	.02	1.7	24.3	0	10
Mashed	1/2 cup	172	.5	.10	2.7	39.8	0	21
Syrup								
Maple,reduced-								
calorie	1 tblsp.	30	.2	0	0	7.8	0	41
Pancake	1 tblsp.	50	0	0	0	12.8	0	2
Tangerine, frsh	1 med.	38	.1	.02	.5	9.6	0	1
Tofu								
Firm	4 ozs	164	9.9	1.43	17.9	4.9	0	16
Soft	4 ozs	60	3	----	7.0	2.0	0	5
Tomato								
Fresh	1 med.	26	.4	.06	1	5.7	0	11
Cooked	1/2 cup	30	.3	.04	1.3	6.8	0	13
Juice, regular	1 cup	41	.1	.02	1.8	10.3	0	881
Juice, no salt	1 cup	41	.1	.02	1.8	10.3	0	24
Paste, regular	1 tblsp.	14	.1	.02	.6	3.1	0	129
Paste, no salt	1 tblsp.	11	0	----	.5	2.6	---	6

FOOD	Serving	Cal.	Fat	S.Fat	Pro	Carb	Cho	Sod
Sauce, regular	1/2 cup	37	.2	.03	1.6	8.8	0	741
Sauce, no salt	1/2 cup	40	0	----	1.2	9.2	---	24
Stewed, canned	1/2 cup	30	1.1	.20	.9	5.2	0	187
Whole, canned, peeled	1/2 cup	22	0	----	.9	5.2	---	424
Whole, canned, no salt	1/2 cup	22	0	----	.9	5.2	---	15

Tortilla

Chips, plain	10 each	135	7.3	1.05	2.1	16	0	24
Corn, 6" round	1 each	67	1.1	.12	2.1	12.8	0	53
Flour, 6" round	1 each	111	23	.56	2.4	22.2	0	0

Turkey, skinned, boned and roasted

White meat	4 ozs	179	3.6	1.16	33.7	0	79	72
Dark meat	4 ozs	212	8.1	2.75	32.4	0	96	89
Smoked	4 ozs	168	6.5	1.93	27.2	0	64	781

Turnip greens,

cooked	1/2 cup	14	.2	.04	.8	3.1	0	21

Turnips,

cooked, cubed	1/2 cup	14	.1	.01	.6	3.8	0	39

Veal, cooked

Ground	4 ozs	195	8.5	3.45	27.6	0	117	95
Leg	4 ozs	171	3.9	1.39	31.9	0	117	77
Loin	4 ozs	199	7.9	2.92	29.9	0	120	109

Vegetable juice cocktail

Regular	1 cup	46	.2	.03	1.5	11	0	883
Low-sodium	1 cup	48	.2	----	2.4	9.7	---	48

Vinegar,

distilled	1 tblsp.	2	0	0	0	.8	0	0

Water chestnuts,

canned, sliced	1/2 cup	35	0	.01	.6	8.7	0	6

Watermelon,

raw, diced	1 cup	51	.7	.35	1	11.5	0	3

Wheat germ	1 tblsp.	26	.7	.12	1.7	3.7	0	1

Whipped cream	1 tblsp.	26	2.8	1.71	.2	.2	10	3

FOOD	Serving	Cal.	Fat	S.Fat	Pro	Carb	Cho	Sod
Whipped topping,								
non-dairy, frozen	1 tblsp.	15	1.2	1.02	0.1	1.1	0	1
Wonton								
wrappers	1 each	6	.1	.03	.2	.9	5	12
Worcestershire sauce								
Regular	1 tblsp.	12	0	0	.3	2.7	0	147
Low-sodium	1 tblsp.	12	0	0	0	3	0	57
Yogurt								
Low-fat	1 cup	193	2.8	1.84	11.2	31.3	11	150
Frozen, low-fat	1/2 cup	99	2	1.41	3	18	10	35
Frozen, nonfat	1/2 cup	82	0	0	3.4	18.1	0	60
Fruit varieties,								
Low-fat	1 cup	225	2.6	1.68	9	42.3	9	120
Plain, low-fat	1 cup	143	3.5	2.27	11.9	16	14	159
Plain, nonfat	1 cup	127	.4	.26	13	17.4	5	173
Zucchini								
Raw	1/2 cup	9	.1	.02	.7	1.9	0	2
Cooked, diced	1/2 cup	17	.1	.01	.7	4.1	0	3

Acknowledgments

Thanks are in order for the U.S. Department of Health and Human Services and to the National Institute of Health, both for their kind contributions of material on cholesterol metabolism. A special thanks is also due to Brian Feinblum, Bryan Silverstein, Vicki Heil and the entire staff at Lifetime Books for their kind help and contributions.

Lifetime Books would like to also give credit to several of its sources: *Cholesterol Cure Made Easy* by Sylvan R. Lewis, M.D. and *The Heart Watcher's Complete Diet and Menu Planner* by Sylvan R. Lewis, M.D.

Nancy Szeman, R.D., would like to give credit to Chef Steven Yacovone of the North Ridge Medical Center in Hollywood, Florida for the following recipes: Eggplant Filled with Mushrooms; Asparagus Risotto; Couscous Salad; Basmati and Wild Rice Salad; and Minted Millet, Cuccumber and Garbanzo Salad.

I would like to give special thanks to cover artist Donna Morris, food photographer Barney Taxel and to my co-author, Nancy Szeman, R.D.

Lastly, I would like to thank Janine Kullman for her diligent and capable help in editing and typing my contribution to the book.

THE TOP 100 RECIPES FOR DIABETICS

Dorothy Kaplan

The Comprehensive Diabetic Cookbook — 3rd Edition.

This comprehensive diabetic cookbook (previous edition sold 60,000 copies) offers over 100 easy-to-prepare nutritionally-sound recipes, including: beef, bread, poultry, fish, veal, fruit & vegetable salads, cheese & eggs, lamb, ground beef, soup, sauces, desserts and beverages.

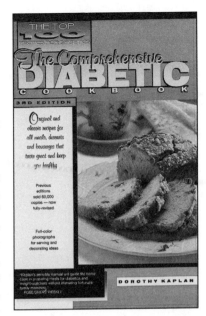

"Diabetes requires proper attention to physical fitness, proper medications and proper nutrition. Dorothy Kaplan's book provides tasty and nutritious foods that meet these requirements. I recommend it highly for diabetic patients."
— **Seymour L. Alterman, M.D., F.A.C.P., Clinical Professor of Medicine and Endocrinology, University of Miami, Florida**

★ *208 pages* ★ *$14.95* ★ *Paperback* ★ *ISBN: 0-8119-0819-4*
★ *Contains 12 color photographs*

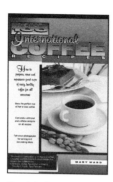

The Top 100 International Coffee Recipes

How to Prepare, Serve and Experience Great Cups of Tasty & Healthy Coffee for All Occasions

Mary Ward

In this beautifully full-colored illustrated book (the perfect gift) you will find one hundred recipes — and trade secrets — for creating the best-tasting, most relaxing and healthiest cup of "black gold."

★ **224 pages with 12 color photos** ★**$14.95**
★**Paperback** ★ **ISBN: 0-8119-0818-6**

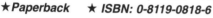

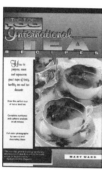

The Top 100 International Tea Recipes

How to Prepare, Serve and Experience Great Cups of Tasty & Healthy Tea and Tea Desserts

Mary Ward

Here is a celebration of original and classic tea recipes. With full-color photographs (the perfect gift) and step-by-step instruction, you will learn the secrets to making the perfect cup of tea.

★ **256 pages with 12 color photos** ★**$14.95**
★**Paperback** ★ **ISBN: 0-8119-0817-8**

Index